Soap, Water, and Sex

Soap, Water, and Sex

A Lively Guide to the Benefits of Sexual Hygiene and to Coping with Sexually Transmitted Diseases

Jacob Lipman, M.D.

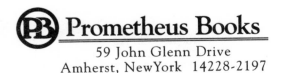

Prometheus Books

59 John Glenn Drive
Amherst, NewYork 14228-2197

Published 1998 by Prometheus Books

01 00 99 98 97   5 4 3 2 1

Library of Congress Cataloging-in-Publication Data

Lipman, Jacob, M.D.
    Soap, water, and sex : a lively guide to the benefits of sexual hygiene and to coping with sexually transmitted diseases / by Jacob Lipman.
        p.   cm.
    Includes bibliographical references and index.
    ISBN 1-57392-193-9 (pbk. : alk. paper)
    1. Hygiene, Sexual. 2. Sexually transmitted diseases. I. Title.
RA788.L57   1997
613.9′5—dc21   97–31405
                                                          CIP

Printed in the United States of America on acid-free paper.

To my wife of forty-seven years, Rita Kenefick Lipman, and her ongoing influence on all the lives she touched as wife, mother, counselor, creative thinker, humanist, and altogether wonderful human being, beautiful in body and spirit.

She died January 8, 1993, at age seventy-seven.

Contents

7

1

Soap, Water, and Sex, Oh, My!

Steve and Maggie were in the middle of a lovers' quarrel. She had just brought him to a climax with her mouth and now demanded to know why he would not reciprocate. The gist of his embarrassed, stumbling reply was that, with bowel movements, urine, vaginal secretions, and menstrual blood all routed through these few secluded inches, he found it difficult to bring his nose and mouth to such a smelly, dirty place.

Surveys have disclosed that many men happily accept fellatio but balk at cunnilingus. Oral-genital practices come highly recommended by numerous sex manuals, are engaged in by a larger number of couples each year, and though it remains against the law in some states, this is not why male partners cringe from satisfying their female counterparts.

We enter love-making anticipating heavenly delights, but, all too often, we encounter a soured earthbound unpleasantness brought on by a failure to cope adequately with some of the byproducts of human bodily functions. Whether or not it occurs during the female menstrual period, intercourse is untidy. The male and female lubricants of sexual arousal mingle with the normal vaginal discharge, and semen, contraceptive jellies and creams, plain commercial lubricants, and saliva may all be mixed in and smeared about by thrusting bodies. On washing, surface conditions are quickly restored to baseline (the precoital state). Unfortunately, for a few of us who are overly finicky and are put off by the initial wetness and the later glued hairs and crusted skin, much of the joy of sexual intercourse fades.

Many of our most underdiscussed, common sexual problems can be prevented or improved—without any help from the popular sex experts Masters and Johnson—using soap, water, a little knowhow, and a few gadgets.

We are living in a vividly unstable era. The political, economic, and social movements in the world have been momentous, and inevitably this has affected relations between the sexes.

Women are increasingly participants in government. More and more they are becoming cobreadwinners with their male partners. In the home and in bed, women are becoming more assertive.

Men also are undergoing role shifts. They are under pressure to accommodate to the evolving women they encounter and to listen attentively to the complaints of the women they live with. They are urged to be more sensitive to a partner's emotional needs and to be more open in sharing their own emotions without worrying that it will result in tarnishing their manly image. Sharing in household chores such as washing dishes, doing the laundry, or diapering the baby is emerging as acceptable male behavior.

A major impact on the sexual behavior of those not involved in a longterm, faithful monogamous relationship has been the modern plague of the past decade or so, the HIV/AIDS epidemic (see chapter 16). AIDS (acquired immunodeficiency syndrome) is a result of an HIV (human immunodeficiency virus) infection. The great usefulness of simple soap and water in coping with HIV infection and many other sexually transmitted diseases will become obvious in the course of this book.

How do soap and water accomplish their good deeds? Mostly by killing all kinds of germs, including bacteria and viruses. A soapy lather allowed to remain on the skin for fifteen seconds will eliminate many germs, because the lather destroys a germ's outer coat, which holds the tiny organism together. This simple precautionary method is rarely discussed in any detail by most books on safer sex. In this book, by contrast, soap and water will be prominently featured as I describe the various steps necessary to ensure safer sex.

The book will also briefly present the various sexually transmitted diseases. Only the most prevalent patterns of each illness are given, because the range of variation among individuals is large. Even in an illness as common as measles, Mary Smith's case may not look at all like John Johnson's case. You will find a description of the nature of the illness, its causation, and its early symptoms and manifestations. The effect of the disease on your sex life and a broad outline of the treatment are given, usually without naming specific medications because some of them may become obsolete practically overnight. Your physician stays abreast of the latest developments in medical practice, so he or she should always be consulted. If you recognize any of the characteristic signs or symptoms of the sexually transmitted diseases in your partner or yourself, early consultation with a physician is stressed. This book should give you enough information to alert you to the need to seek professional help.

The book concludes with a short but meaningful summary, plus a glossary of technical terms, bibliography of recommended reading, and an index.

2

Odors: A Common Problem

A bundant literature on mouth odors is available to the public, but discussion of anogenital odors and what to do about them is not so readily accessible. Such odors, however, can be one of the biggest sexual turn-offs. There is no shortage of pussyfooting media advertisements for scented, odor-masking products, and in drug stores and supermarkets the shelves are full of the related douche and spray displays. However, honest, dependable explanations of the causes of those odors and proper advice on how to remedy them are not easy to find. There need be no disagreeable odors about the vulva and anus, any more than there are about the elbow, if the proper care is provided.

Unless a woman has just bathed, there will be an odor of urine about the vulva. When the urine exits the urethra—the short passage leading from the urinary bladder to the outside world—it flows over the inner surface of the labia, the vulval lips, rinsing away some of the naturally accumulating vaginal secretions and wetting some of the genital hairs. Wiping with toilet tissue will not remove it all. Over the hours, the bacteria which are always present on body surfaces act to produce a stale urine odor. Because most American homes and public toilet facilities do not have bidets, bathroom fixtures that spray water over the anal-vaginal region to cleanse it more thoroughly, this odor remains a fact of life.

Men are not exempt from this same type of odor. After urinating, the male urethra—which is eight or nine inches long to the female's one-and-a-half inches—still holds about a teaspoonful of urine. The customary few seconds of shaking the penis above a urinal may dislodge a few drops, but never all of the liquid. The penis is replaced in the underpants, and, over the next minute or two, the rest of the teaspoonful is deposited on the underwear. By the end of the day, an odorous, yellow stain has appeared on the shorts. In addition, during urination some of the urine may back up under the foreskin of uncircumcised males, creating an additional odor problem.

Both men and women may suffer from odors originating in the anal region. Wiping certainly does not remove all feces and its odor; smears of stool may remain, especially if there is considerable hairiness or if there are tags of skin resulting from hemorrhoids. Careful washing is required to remove these traces.

More complicated odor problems result from vaginal discharges, which are an unavoidable part of every woman's life. Between the menstrual periods, a small amount of mucuslike fluid oozes from the vagina, so that by the end of the day the crotch of the panties may have a yellowish, greenish, or brownish stain and an odor. This vaginal discharge is normal, induced by hormone stimulation of the vagina, and it is not a sign of infection. The discharge is not considered excessive if the individual is not conscious of wetness and if the panties do not require changing more than once a day.

The chief female hormone, estrogen, has a maturing effect on the lining of the vagina, causing the topmost of the three layers of cells in the lining to constitute 90 to 95 percent of the cells present. These superficial cells, as they are known, contain large amounts of starch. Of the bacteria and yeast normally inhabiting the vagina, the Döderlein bacillus plays an important part in keeping the vagina healthy by fermenting the starch in superficial cells into a fluid with acid properties. This acidity helps keep the vagina healthy by producing an environment hostile to many foreign organisms that may cause an inflammation of the vagina. If the Döderlein bacilli are killed off by antibiotics given for an infection elsewhere in the body, the vagina may become less acid and allow the yeast residing there to proliferate into a symptom-causing yeast infection.

An increased vaginal discharge, sometimes pro-

nouncedly malodorous, may result from a variety of factors, such as infection, irritation, or even sexual excitement, and it may cause redness and itching of the vulva,
soreness on wiping, or a burning felt on contact with
urine. The current practice of wearing panty hose plus
slacks or jeans also interferes with the evaporation of
moisture from the vulva, in which case the normal
vaginal discharge may give rise to inflammation. A persistent increase of vaginal discharge or persistent irritation is a signal to seek professional help. (Menstruation,
perhaps the most widely acknowledged form of vaginal
discharge, and cleanliness of the vaginal region will be
discussed in the next chapter.)

There are zones other than those commonly considered erogenous where soap and water may be used to
enhance sexual attractiveness. Usually a body that has
just become sweaty radiates an honest, earthy odor, but
when the skin bacteria act by the hour on dead, sweat-
moistened cells, cells that are endlessly shed by the skin,
a disagreeable odor of decay may result. This is particularly so wherever sweat may not have a chance to evap-
orate: the overhanging abdomen of a particularly stout
person may rest on the pubis or groin, while in women
of quite average build the underside of the breasts press
against the chest, and for most of us there are places on
our bodies where skin folds remain in contact with each
other. The odor of putrefaction that develops after
sweating may not be noticed by the offending individual, because a persistent odor quickly tires the sense
of smell into unawareness. Frequent and conscientious

washing and drying between surfaces in contact with each other, especially in warm weather, as between the toes, or even under the free edge of the toenails, will keep the slender, as well as the overweight, safer from unwelcome odor.

Odors: Sexual Turn-On

All this discussion of odors makes it sound as though everyone is turned off by the natural unprocessed emanations of the body, but that is not so. The same "bad" odors that repel certain individuals create erotic excitement in others. This is because the sense of smell is important in exciting sexual desire. As it does in animals, loss of the sense of smell lowers the sex drive of human beings.

Many men find the scent of normal vaginal secretions very attractive. Scientists believe this may be due to the existence in those secretions of pheromones, chemical substances produced in animals that even in tiny amounts evoke a strong physical response in other animals of the same species. For example, it's the pheromone emitted by the bitch in heat that provokes the local population of male dogs to cluster about her. Scientists are investigating whether human males are also responsive to that kind of sexual stimulus.

Of course we have for centuries used substances that filled the role of providing stimulating scents to attract a male. We call them perfumes. But remember that perfumes are designed for their fragrance and not for their flavor. They taste terrible! Therefore, they are best not applied where a mouth may be placed.

3

Cleanliness How-To's

A special case of increased vaginal flow is the menstrual period, which occurs about monthly in a normal woman before menopause if she has not become pregnant. Each month, after shedding most of the lining of the uterus, which had been prepared to receive and nourish a fertilized egg, the overripe lining passes out as the menstrual flow, or menses. Ordinarily sanitary napkins (also called pads) and vaginal tampons are used to absorb the menses.

There are certain disadvantages to the use of pads: Their bulk may be visible through close-fitting apparel; they may chafe; and they require frequent changing to prevent the development of an offensive odor. For these reasons, many women prefer to use tampons rather than pads. Tampons are inserted into the vagina, and therefore they are not visible. The tampon wearer is not conscious of its presence. They cause no chafing and odor is less likely to be a problem, but they do have their own disadvantages.

One such "disadvantage" is the possibility of toxic shock syndrome, a life-threatening condition that may affect tampon users (but which also hits nonusers, and even males, as well). This condition has brought into serious question the safety of allowing a single tampon to remain in place for eight hours or more. Some physicians now recommend that tampons be removed at least every four to six hours and that an external pad be worn during sleep. Many other doctors now consent to overnight use of our current tampons, i.e., for eight hours.

Toxic shock syndrome made headlines in 1980 with about seven hundred cases reported, most associated with tampon use. The symptoms and signs included sudden onset with fever, headache, sore throat, vomiting, watery diarrhea, tiredness, confusion off and on, and a rash resembling sunburn. Very low blood pressure developed in a day or two. Between 8 and 15 percent of the severely ill patients died. Highly absorbent tampons that were on the market at the time were later removed when it was suspected that their high absorbency might in some way promote the growth of the staphylococci that were the usual organisms producing the poison that caused the toxic shock syndrome. Toward the end of the first week of illness peeling of the skin occurred in some patients, sometimes of the fingertips or the hands, but sometimes over large areas of the body.

A number of women will "lose" a tampon in the vagina. The depths of the vagina being rather insensitive, the presence of a foreign body, even one as large as a tampon, evokes no sensation once it is in place. If, in the act of insertion, the string attached to the tampon to facilitate its later withdrawal is pushed into the vagina with the tampon, or if the string becomes detached from the tampon, it is easy to forget that a tampon is present. In a matter of days such a forgotten tampon will assess its disagreeable penalty for the forgetfulness: a foul discharge which will last until the tampon is removed.

Occasionally, cuplike rubber or plastic inserts are used to catch the menstrual flow. These are removed, emptied, washed, and reinserted as necessary, frequently if the flow is heavy. A contraceptive diaphragm may also be used in this way. (By sequestering the bloody flow in the upper vagina, a diaphragm is particularly useful in reducing the messiness of intercourse during a menstrual period.)

These "damming" methods have to be used cautiously, particularly with a heavy menstrual flow, when the dam should be emptied frequently. If the accumulating blood is allowed to build up a pressure, it may back into the uterus, through the fallopian tubes, and into the abdominal cavity which is lined by a thin membrane known as the peritoneum. The blood irritates the lining, causing a painful inflammation, peritonitis.

Some doctors believe that endometriosis, another

painful condition, may also result from menses backing up through the fallopian tubes. The bits of uterine tissue contain small clumps of viable cells. If these back up through the fallopian tubes, they find a warm, moist, favorable intra-abdominal environment. Some of these clumps of living cells, derived from the lining of the uterus, thrive on the outer surface of the tubes, the ovaries, the uterus, the urinary bladder, the intestine, the liver, and so forth. Being living cells, they multiply and, just as the lining cells of the uterus do, under the influence of the female hormones, estrogen and progesterone, they undergo the same cyclic changes that the cells lining the uterus do. Parts of the nodule of cells are shed at the time of menstruation with bleeding. Blood is very irritating to the peritoneum. Therefore, each month a "chemical" peritonitis occurs, not caused by germs but by the irritant effects of the red blood cells. The inflammation of the peritoneum may lead to severe abdominal pain and tenderness with difficulty moving about because of the pain. These recurrent bouts of inflammation lead to intra-abdominal adhesions and other complications.

Hormone pills can be used to turn off the menstrual cycles and there will be no further shedding of blood within the abdominal cavity and, as a result, a cessation of monthly bouts of severe abdominal pain. Sometimes the adhesions may lead to bowel obstruction and other conditions that may require surgery.

Douching

For some women, another source of distress during sex is the odor of putrefaction that may develop from blood shed on the last days of the menstrual period. Fresh blood is essentially odorless, but blood that stagnates for six or eight hours during the night or for several hours while a woman is sitting in a chair can produce an odor of putrefaction caused by the action of bacteria in the vagina. Does this call for douching? Not really. Douching is not a must, because, given time, the healthy vagina will cleanse itself, gravity removing the source of the odor. However, if a sexual encounter is imminent, or if self-assurance is promoted by it, then a douche is worthwhile.

A woman in normal health need never douche. In abnormal conditions, douching is best done on professional advice, and the kind of douche and the frequency of douching are prescribed. (One commonly used solution is made with two tablespoonfuls of white vinegar to each quart of lukewarm tap water.) Also, it is advisable to get professional recommendations before using any over-the-counter feminine hygiene products, such as commercial douche preparations. Some of the vaginal douche powders and liquids are intrinsically irritating; some of the products may cause allergic reactions; and some are alkaline (the normal vagina is an acid environment). Changing the vagina's degree of acidity allows disease-causing bacteria to flourish.

For women who have never douched, the process

seems formidable but is really quite simple. Douching, typically, is done using a two-quart plastic or rubber reservoir whose contents flow out through a length of tubing with a nozzle at the end. The nozzle has holes along the sides but not at the tip. The flow is controlled in on-and-off fashion by a clip on the tubing. The reservoir is hung so the bottom of the bag is no more than one foot above the level of the entrance to the vagina. (Hanging the bag too high may produce enough pressure to force the fluid into the uterus. Fluid forced into the uterus may continue through the fallopian tubes and create a peritonitis with the bacteria washed from the vagina.) The douche may be taken sitting on the toilet or lying in the bathtub. The nozzle is introduced deeply into the vagina, the labia are pressed around the nozzle where it enters the vagina in order to prevent the immediate outflow of the cleansing liquid, and then the clip is opened. When the vagina feels distended, the clip is released, and the solution is allowed to flow out of the vagina. The process is repeated until the reservoir is empty.

Some women will douche after sexual intercourse to ease their worry about getting pregnant. In other words, they may rely on douching as a form of birth control. However, this is not an effective method of preventing pregnancy, because the douching solution must contact the sperm directly to destroy them, something which is difficult to ensure. Sperm begin swimming toward the cervix and uterus within seconds of ejaculation, and no matter how quickly a woman douches after intercourse, by the time she does, many sperm have already passed through the cervix out of reach of the douching solution.

Douching equipment, intended for bathing the vagina, is easily contaminated, and for that reason should never be used for taking an enema or lent to others.

A douche should not be performed a full day before a pelvic examination. This is because one of the reasons physicians perform such exams is to see the vagina and cervix as they are usually, not freshly washed.

Washing the Genital Area

Without careful washing of the external genitals, for women the daily normal vaginal discharge plus the oily products of the skin's sebaceous glands can lead to malodorous, caked accumulations between the labia minora and labia majora (the inner and outer lips of the vulva) and in other folds and crevices. Urination washes away some of the build up, but more than just cursory bathing is required to remove the rest.

Fearing their little girls might discover the pleasures of genital friction and masturbate, some mothers leave cleansing of the genital area to a soak in the tub or a quick splash of water. As adults, some of their daughters remain too hasty in washing that region to do a thorough job. Just as the ears call for special attention in bathing, so does the vulva.

Arguments can be made in favor of both tub bathing

and showering as the "better" way to get oneself clean. In general, the women in my medical practice tended to favor taking a bath, and the men preferred a shower. A tub bath can be leisurely and restful, and the vulval and anal regions are immersed in water, which may provide a more thorough cleansing, whereas these areas are protected from direct contact with the spray in a shower unless a movable shower head is used. On the other hand, without a rinse afterward, a tub bath may leave a soapy residue which is normally washed away during the course of a shower.

There remains one infrequently mentioned potential source of vulval odor, the clitoris. There are still many women (and men) unaware that women also have the equivalent of a penis. Except for the size difference, and the fact that there is no outlet for urine located at the tip of the clitoris, penis and clitoris are similar structures.

Fathers teach uncircumcised boys to pull back the foreskin to expose and wash away the cheesy grayish or yellowish coatings of smegma that are constantly being produced under the foreskin, as long-standing collections of smegma may cause inflammation and a foul odor. Smegma contains fat, cellular debris, and keratin (a chief structural material of hair and nails). Girls have a foreskin, too, but very few mothers teach their daughters to retract the foreskin of the clitoris when bathing, or show them how to deal in other ways with the debris that may have accumulated under the clitoral foreskin.

The recess between the foreskin and the head of the clitoris is a blind alley entirely lined by skin. In some women the recess is so shallow that ordinary bathing removes all the smegma, and in others retraction of the foreskin gives sufficient exposure for thorough cleansing. For some women, however, the recess is deep, or the foreskin cannot be pulled back, and, for them, probing gently with a cotton-tipped swab moistened with water is a safe and usually effective procedure. Such cleansing should be done at regular intervals. Adhesions between the foreskin and the head of the clitoris will interfere with smegma removal in a few individuals, who may wish to consult with a physician about the problem. These are usually very thin strands from the clitoris to the prepuce. If some of the adhesions don't permit cleansing with a moistened cotton swab, a physician should be seen to "break" the adhesion so that cleansing can be properly done.

Men have an advantage here in the mobility and direct visibility of the penis. Many women cannot see their clitoris directly, fixed as it is at the lower underside of the pubic region. A mirror and a properly placed light may have to be used to remove the smegma satisfactorily.

Anal Intercourse and Cleanliness

Just as individuals differ in their response to any given odor, so, too, do they differ in their feelings about anal sexual activity. Although generally recognized as a major erogenous zone, for many the anus is esthetically

and otherwise unacceptable as an arena for sexual pleasure. For some people, though, it is a prime resource for
the giving and receiving of sexual gratification. According to the findings in the statistically most reliable
sex survey done in the United States to date,* rectal
intercourse, although illegal in many states, has been
tried at least once by 26 percent of males and 20 percent
of females. Passive anal intercourse was not at all
appealing to 87 percent of women and 79 percent of
men, and active anal intercourse was not at all appealing
to 78 percent of men.

Oral-anal sex, anilingus, calls for more than ordinary
preparatory fastidiousness. Even under virtually anti-
septic conditions, however, putting the tongue to the
anal region may lead to an old-fashioned venereal disease in a stylishly new location (such as syphilis on the
tongue or gonorrhea of the throat) or to such nasty illnesses as hepatitis, assorted dysenteries, or the itchy
nuisance of a pinworm infestation.

Because so many people experiment with anal intercourse, and many practice it extensively, it is important
to discuss its risks and discomforts, which can be
reduced through proper care. Feces that may become
smeared externally or block entry—obvious drawbacks
—may be emptied from the rectum by an enema before
sex takes place. Sexual excitement may lubricate the
vagina and cause drops of slippery fluid to appear at the

*Robert Michael et al., *Sex in America* (Boston: Little,
Brown & Co., 1994), pp. 140–47.

tip of the penis, but the anus stays dry. Therefore, insertion is difficult or impossible without the application of a lubricant such as K-Y® Jelly, petroleum jelly, mineral oil, contraceptive jelly, saliva, etc. If a condom is being used, only water-soluble solutions should be used, as will be discussed in detail in the next chapter.

Pain and bleeding may result if the anal canal is narrow and unable to stretch as much as the penis requires. The anal canal and rectum are easily damaged, so that vigorous thrusting may tear the anal or rectal wall, causing hemorrhage or a serious local infection. The blood of an HIV carrier is a very effective transmitter of an HIV infection. The human immunodeficiency virus (which causes AIDS), gonorrhea, and other infections can be transferred via penis to rectum, or from rectum to penis.

If anal intercourse immediately precedes an approach to the vulva or vagina, both hands and penis should be washed thoroughly with soap to minimize the chances of introducing infection into the female genital tract.

Hair: Sexy or Not?

Getting back to sexual attractiveness, is a man more sexy shaved or bearded, furry-bodied or almost hairless? Is hair in the armpit of a woman unattractive, or is it sexually provocative?

In general, American women shave their armpits but

do not touch the pubic region, but there are cultures abroad, and subcultures in America, in which shaving the pubis and vulva are high style. Shaving the legs is not as popular in other parts of the world as it is in this country. In the United States, before a woman delivered her baby, it had been the practice of most hospitals to shave the pubic region, the labia majora, and adjacent thighs, often with later complaints of itching and prickling as the hair grew back. Women who are distressed by coarse hairs on breasts or chin may shave them, or pluck them out, or have them removed in other ways.

Men express their own individuality as well as membership in a given subculture through distinctive hair styles. Walk down any main street and you'll encounter some beards shaved into artistic patterns and others untouched by comb or brush for years; moustaches, long or short, turned up or turned down; and, mostly, the clean or almost clean shaven. A stroll on the beach will disclose an occasional shaved chest. Competitive swimmers often shave their entire bodies to reduce drag in the water. Statistics on pubic-hair shaving in men, however, are hard to come by.

We'll all have to wait for scientific studies to resolve the effect of these various hair styles on sexual success, or lack of it.

4

Your Good Friend, the Condom

When it comes to sexual hygiene, soap and water have a great ally in the condom. The condom is not worn nearly often enough, even by those people fully aware of its usefulness. It is widely used for birth control, but even there it is too often neglected. "I don't like to use them, because they cut down on sensation!" is the reason most often given for failing to use a condom. We have to pay a price for certain advantages we wish to enjoy in life, and reduced sensation seems like a real bargain compared to the unwanted pregnancy or venereal disease that the condom may prevent. As a welcome fringe benefit of its use, the reduced sensitivity may actually allow the pleasure of the act of intercourse to be prolonged.

The condom provides excellent protection to both sexes against many sexually transmitted diseases, including infection from HIV, the cause of the AIDS, which remains at disastrously epidemic levels worldwide. Any of us who play the field sexually may encounter individuals infected with a venereal disease of which they are unaware but which they are capable of transmitting to others. The penile sores of syphilis or chancroid or herpes (all of which will be detailed later in this book) may be inconspicuous or mistaken for the result of a chance injury (such as an abrasion from intercourse or a small laceration from a fingernail). Gonorrhea may mark time in the urethra or in the vagina without calling attention to itself by causing a discharge. The vagina may harbor a number of venereal diseases without displaying give-away signs or symptoms. There are also plenty of people among us who are unscrupulous enough to engage in sexual intercourse fully aware that they are infected.

It is sound and possibly lifesaving advice that—unless you have been faithful in your marriage or long-term relationship—a condom should always be used during intercourse, whether vaginal or rectal, or in fellatio, the incidence of sexually transmitted disease being as high as it is.

The condom, most often a sheath of very thin latex, open at one end and designed to fit over the erect penis, is a marvelous invention that provides a measure of safety for couples acting responsibly in this era's hazardous sexual environment.

Condoms made from animal intestine, "skins," are

preferred by many for the almost condom-free sensations they allow during intercourse, but unfortunately
skins have tiny pores in their walls that do not prevent
the passage of even tinier viruses (such as HIV, herpes,
and wart virus), making skins unsuitable for disease
prevention. Some researchers have tried to develop
plastic condoms, but those that were tried broke too
easily. New, stronger versions made of polyurethane
should appear on the market, but the effectiveness of
such condoms, according to the Food and Drug Administration, is currently unknown.*

At a cost ranging from about twenty-five cents to
more than a dollar each, condoms can be bought at drug
stores, some supermarkets, from dispensers in public
toilets, or by mail. The armed forces hand them out free
to their personnel, as do some schools to their students.

Condoms are usually rolled up in a sealed plastic or
foil package, but some come flat and unrolled. Most are
about seven inches long by about two inches wide, but a
few come in other sizes. Some are transparent; some are
colored; some have a reservoir tip (a nipplelike projec-
tion at the closed end to receive the ejaculate); some have
a thinner wall than others (it should be noted, however,
that the thickness of latex condoms varies only by hun-
dredths of a millimeter); some are contoured for a
snugger fit; some are lubricated; some have a contraceptive chemical coating (most often nonoxynol-9 which,

---

*"How Reliable Are Condoms?" *Consumer Reports* (May
1995): 320–25.

especially in the higher concentrations found in some contraceptive jellies, may act as an anti-infective agent against some sexually transmitted diseases); and some are ribbed, that is, covered with small bumps, presumably to enhance female pleasure. It would be a good idea to try a variety of condoms to determine which prove most satisfactory.

A condom for females made of polyurethane, which covers the vulva and lines the vagina, recently entered the marketplace. The reliability and usefulness of the female condom await large scale experience with it.

Unless used properly, a condom may prove to be of little or no value, but condoms made or sold in the United States are highly reliable when properly stored and used. Prolonged exposure to heat, even that within a wallet or a car's glove compartment, may cause the latex to degrade, so supplies should be kept in a cool place, such as the medicine chest or bedside table. Oil-based materials, such as petroleum jelly, also weaken latex, and should therefore never be used as lubricants with condoms. If a lubricant is required, a water-based one, such as K-Y® Jelly, should be used. Extended exposure to water also deteriorates rubber. Also, be advised that if the condom's package is not intact, the condom should not be used, since it could have deteriorated or punctured. Condoms should be used only once and then discarded; each act of intercourse calls for a fresh condom.

In the United States, condom failure is rarely due to manufacturing imperfections, but the reliability of condoms manufactured in certain other parts of the world cannot be counted on. Failures which occur in American-made condoms usually result from improper use or storage. Therefore, if you are going abroad, it might be wise to take a stock of condoms with you and be certain to store and use them correctly.

A condom should be applied as soon as erection occurs, certainly before the penis is seriously engaged. There is a lubricating fluid generated by Cowper's glands, which leaks from the penis in most men shortly after the onset of sexual arousal. This fluid may contain HIV and other organisms capable of causing a sexually transmitted disease. There may even be some sperm in Cowper's secretion.

Because the package holding the condom may be difficult to open without scissors, rehearsing the process before the need arises may prevent untimely awkwardness. In fact, it is a good idea for first-time users to read the directions in the package and practice putting on a condom before they try to use one during sex. The practice condom should then be properly disposed of. Some men feel that interrupting foreplay to put the condom on is an objectionable feature of condom use, but practice will provide the skill necessary to reduce or avoid any discomfort. If the wearer's partner becomes involved in helping put on the condom, then foreplay may even be enhanced.

The condom is placed on the head of the penis, after the foreskin (if it is present) has been pulled back. If the condom has no reservoir tip, about a half inch of the end of the condom is pinched flat as the condom is unrolled down to the base of the penis, to provide space for the ejaculate. Care should be taken not to trap air under the condom along the way. Air trapped in the condom may cause it to burst with the explosive addition of ejaculate.

Some users put a small amount of slippery contraceptive jelly or other water-soluble lubricant in the closed end of the condom before donning it so that in thrusting the condom slides on the penis, heightening the pleasurable sensations of intercourse, but that's a risky practice. Unlike lubricated condoms, which are evenly lubricated to avoid slippage, lubricant applied only at the tip may work its way up the length of the penis and the condom may slip off. Even without this added lubricant within the condom, the male's natural lubricating fluid that leaks from the penis during sexual excitement may be profuse enough during prolonged intercourse to result in the condom slipping off.

Sometimes the vagina lacks enough natural lubricant for intercourse to proceed comfortably. In such a case a water-soluble artificial substitute, such as a contraceptive jelly, or K-Y® Jelly, may be applied to the entrance to or deep within the vagina, or to the outside surface of the condom. With the use of the lubricant the condom is less likely to break as a result of friction, an upsetting event that occurs about once in a hundred episodes of sexual intercourse.

Contraceptive Jellies

Like condoms, contraceptive jellies may be purchased over the counter at most pharmacies and some grocery stores. Contraceptive (i.e., spermicidal) creams are also available, but as these tend to be oil-based, they are not suitable for use with latex condoms. (Contraceptive jellies are often used in conjunction with diaphragms and cervical caps.) It is a good idea, when a contraceptive jelly is first purchased, to buy a package with an applicator enclosed. That way only the tube of jelly will need to be replaced.

The applicator is a long, straight plastic tube that screws onto the same threads as the cap that closes the tube. Squeezing jelly into the applicator forces the plunger, which fits snugly into the barrel of the applicator, almost to the top of the applicator, which is then unscrewed from the tube and gently inserted into the vagina as far as it will go and then withdrawn about an inch. The plunger is then depressed until the entire contents of the applicator are deposited in the vagina. The applicator and plunger should always be washed with soap and water after use.

If rectal use is planned, a separate tube of jelly and another applicator are needed to prevent introducing germs from the anus and rectum into the vagina, which might occur if the rectal applicator were not adequately cleaned.

It has been found that in laboratory tests, nonoxynol-9, the sperm-killing chemical in most contraceptive jellies, destroys the organisms causing gonorrhea, syphilis, HIV infections, herpes, and other sexually transmitted diseases. Only with respect to gonorrhea and chlamydia infections in actual emergencies have the results corroborated the findings in test tubes. Spermicides have not yet been tested for their effectiveness in preventing infections following rectal intercourse.

Except in the case where no other contraceptive or prophylactic devices are available, spermicides should never be used alone. Instead, they should always be used in conjunction with some barrier method, such as a diaphragm or condom.

After ejaculation the penis must be removed from the vagina well before it shrinks back to its flaccid state to avoid slippage of the condom and spillage of the ejaculate. Even so, the fingers should be used to hold the condom firmly on the base of the penis during the withdrawal to assure that the condom does not slip off and undo the benefits of its use.

After careful removal from the penis, the condom should be observed for tears or leaks (small leaks will show up on filling the condom with water), and then discarded in the garbage. If there has been a tear or leak, or if the condom slipped off during intercourse, two applicatorsful of contraceptive jelly (containing nonoxynol-9 or an equivalent chemical) should immediately be inserted deep in the vagina to reduce the chance of pregnancy or infection. For safeguarding the mouth from the vulva or anus, or vice versa, a germ-impervious barrier similar to the condom stretched across the entire space between the contacting parts permits the erotic oral stimulation to proceed in safety. Plastic wrap may be used as such a barrier, as may a rubber dam used by dentists, or, using scissors, a suitable sheet of thin rubber may be fashioned from a large latex surgical glove. These measures act similarly to the condom in preventing the transfer of disease organisms between partners.

Any areas of the body that have contacted any of a partner's body fluids should be thoroughly washed with soap and water, allowing the latter to remain in contact with the skin for at least fifteen seconds because any contact with infected body fluids may be dangerous. (Soap destroys germs by breaking down their enveloping wall.) Syphilis, herpes, and possibly HIV may pass through perfectly normal unbroken mucous membranes. Even a tiny abrasion or cut in the skin, such as that which may result from the friction of intercourse, may allow the virus responsible for AIDS through as well as the causative organisms of other sexually transmitted diseases.

5

Thrills, Chills, Perils, and Some Sound Advice

So far in this book I have dealt mostly with matters that have no great bearing on long-term health or lifespan, but I have touched very briefly on some serious conditions such as gonorrhea, syphilis, and AIDS, which can be devastating, even fatal.

When I was in medical school more than fifty years ago, the textbooks listed five venereal diseases: granuloma inguinale, lymphogranuloma venereum, chancroid, gonorrhea, and syphilis. Now we recognize about thirty, the exact number depending on how strictly the criteria applied are used for defining diseases as "sexually transmitted." Are they transmitted sexually often, or at least occasionally? May different organisms offer up

41

the same picture of disease? In the early developmental stages of sexually transmitted diseases, one disease my be mistaken for another, such as chancroid being mistaken for a syphilitic chancre. Also, with respect to bacterial vaginosis, there has been, and continues to be, uncertainty as to which organism, or combination of organisms, is responsible for a given case.

Because sexually transmitted diseases (STDs) have become so prevalent, if those of us who are sexually active outside a long-standing, faithful marriage or relationship wish to remain healthy, we must know how to recognize and cope with the hazards in the community.

Avoidance of all sexual contact with others is an obvious way to improve your chances of not getting a sexually transmitted disease, but many of us would rather not live lives of abstinence. When it comes to sex, many pressures drive our choices but, in the end, those choices remain up to us to make individually. As social animals, we like being with others. As sexual creatures, we require a certain amount of skin-to-skin touching, body-to-body contact with others to remain contented. Just as we crave food when we're hungry, we also crave sexual gratification. But filling our social and sexual needs is no simple matter. All sorts of difficulties get in the way: religious, legal, and financial considerations, among others, and, more concretely, fear of pregnancy and of sexually transmitted diseases. Living in emotional and physical good health while operating within the limits of morality, conscience, prudence, and a host of other factors is no easy job. To make the choices a little easier without completely frustrating our need for a good life, the rest of this book will narrow its focus to the sexually transmitted diseases.

We must know the dangers lurking in the sexual landscape and what to do about them.

Safer Sex: How to Get Started

Step 1

Now let's see what's involved in making sex safer. Let's assume you've just met very attractive Michael, or Helen, and quickly filed him or her in your mind as a potential sex partner.

Being a normally cautious person, you unobtrusively check for undesirable traits: World-class bore? Maniacally jealous? Hair-trigger mood swings? Such a rough screening is nowhere near enough, however. For your mutual protection you need to know more about each other quickly.

In our present forbidding sexual climate, the questions requiring favorable answers will almost certainly prove to be embarrassments for both of you, but asking them is a must. It takes considerable courage for people who have only recently met to initiate such a frank exchange, especially since the initiator must operate on the bold assumption that the other person is also interested in a possible sexual relationship.

To keep things simple, in this scenario Helen will be

the questioner—because of the added risk of pregnancy, with which the male need not concern himself, the female has considerably more at stake. Also, women have more reasons than men do for dreading sexually transmitted diseases. Men, with their more conspicuous, accessible, external anatomy, are more likely to notice the early changes induced by venereal diseases and may therefore seek medical attention before major damage results. Women, victimized by long-hidden, silent attacks, probably suffer more than their share of catastrophic developments, such as sterility, as a result of sexually transmitted diseases.

Helen, before starting to ask Michael questions, will have been concerned with her own personal list of questions:

> Will he be upset when I bring these things up, or will he be grateful that I bring into the open what he's concerned about, too?
>
> Will he assume from my familiarity with AIDS and sexually transmitted diseases that I've been promiscuous?
>
> Does he dislike women taking the initiative in anything sexual?

And so on.

Helen will have made up her mind that her first duty to herself is to remain healthy physically and emotionally. She is also aware that the appeal of sexual pleasure would fade rapidly if she had to worry about getting pregnant or about the long-term effects of sexually transmitted diseases on her fertility, or the fear of a miserable death from AIDS. Contraception and avoidance of sexually transmitted diseases must always rank among her highest concerns in any newly entered sexual encounter.

For their relationship to flourish, Michael and Helen would have to minimize risk for each other as well as for themselves. For example, Michael's failure to agree to use a condom in each act of intercourse or fellatio, or to take any other precautions Helen felt necessary for her peace of mind should send her elsewhere for a sexual partner.

The questions that must be asked can't be posed out of the blue. They require considerable thought for their introduction and shaping and a broad knowledge of HIV and the other sexually transmitted diseases, including how to avoid catching them.

The dialogue that develops as the questions and answers unfold may move in all sorts of directions, and concrete, factual awareness helps validate the coarse probing into the couple's most private past.

Helen might introduce her questioning this way:

"Michael, I find myself attracted to you, but before I allow myself to get closer to you I have to keep a promise I made to myself. In this time of spreading AIDS and other venereal diseases, I will try not to get involved with anyone likely to disturb my physical and emotional health. For these conditions to be met, we really have to know a lot about each other before interacting physically. I can feel my face turning red as I say it!"

Encouraged by Michael's response, Helen would be emboldened to go on and ask the following questions:

- Are you married?
- Have you ever had herpes, gonorrhea, syphilis, or any other venereal diseases?
- Have you been tested for HIV, the virus that causes AIDS?
- Have any of your partners ever tested positive?
- How many sex partners have you had? Did any of these have a lot of sex partners?
- Do you ever go to a prostitute?
- Are you hetero-, homo-, or bisexual?
- Have you ever injected yourself with drugs? Have you ever had a lover who had used intravenous drugs?
- Was a condom used every time you had sex?

Helen has good reasons for asking these questions. For example:

- Getting involved with a married individual is universally recognized as "asking for trouble."
- Association with prostitutes, intravenous drug users or gay men, all groups with notoriously high levels of HIV infection, would place Michael low on her appropriate-candidate list.
- The more sex partners any person has had the more likely it is that that person is carrying a sexually transmitted disease.

Some questions might be based on these scary statistics:

Genital herpes is estimated to be present in over thirty million Americans, and the genital wart virus is believed present in roughly the same number. At present, there is no cure for these viral infections, and condoms provide only limited protection against them. In 1993, fifty-six million Americans were reckoned by health authorities to have at least one sexually transmitted disease, with about three million new cases reported annually. Since only certain sexually transmitted diseases must be reported to the health authorities, many other cases never get counted.

The Associated Press recently conducted a telephone survey using as its subjects one thousand randomly selected women between the ages of eighteen and sixty.* Some of the women said they were informed on AIDS, but two-thirds of the women knew "little or nothing" about sexually transmitted diseases, a surprising disclosure from sexually active individuals. Equally surprising, about three-quarters of the women under age twenty-five who had had many sex partners, many of whom themselves had had extensive sexual experience, were not concerned about contracting sexually transmitted diseases, an amazing indifference.

Many women, and fewer men, infected with a sexually transmitted disease may display no symptoms that would indicate to them or to a partner that they are

---

*See editorial in the *New York Times,* April 7, 1993

capable of infecting someone with any of a number of sexually transmitted diseases, including an HIV infection.

Women, in general, pick up sexually transmitted diseases more readily than men and may suffer more severe consequences. Men, with the easy visibility of the outlet of the urinary passage and the surface of the penis, can notice painless discharges or penile sores early in their development. Women, with their much less easily visible vulva and hidden vagina and cervix, will not be aware of painless urinary-tract discharges that mingle with their vaginal discharge or of painless vaginal and cervical lesions. Also, a premenopausal woman, having a normal daily discharge from the vagina, may be unaware of a slight increase of the discharge and therefore she may not realize that she has acquired a new illness. The genital anatomy of men gives them an early-alert system for a number of sexually transmitted diseases. Many germs prefer a damp, warm environment, such as the vagina or cervix, over the dry surface of a penis. The longer a venereal disease remains undetected the more damage it can do. A woman having a single unprotected act of sexual intercourse with a gonorrhea-infected man stands at least a 50 percent chance of catching it. By contrast, only 20 percent of men will contract gonorrhea after having a single episode of unprotected sex with a gonorrhea-infected woman.

Because some sexually transmitted diseases are more difficult to diagnose in women than in men, and because unnoticed, undiagnosed inapparent infections are more common in women, long-term personal tragedies may result, including infertility, spontaneous abortion, ectopic pregnancy and its complications, diseased babies, and, for the women themselves, the possibility of a shortened lifespan.

The average American has about six or seven sex partners in a lifetime, and each of these, in turn, has about sex or seven. It's a fact of life that the more sexual partners you have the more likely you are to pick up a sexually transmitted disease, or a few sexually transmitted diseases, since it's also a fact that multiple sexually transmitted diseases can be picked up in a single sexual encounter. Also, having a sexually transmitted disease makes it easier to pick up additional venereal diseases including infection with HIV, because open sores from one disease are likely to be infected by another.

That's enough of statistics for now, but the numbers and the rates are important to remember.

Since sexual histories are frequently embellished on the one hand or far too sketchy on the other, it's safer for both partners to have reservations about trusting the information given. No matter how sparkling clean the past and present Michael or Helen appears, it's safer for them to treat each other as high-risk candidates and use all the indicated safer sex precautions for at least six months. (It's not unusual for it to take that long to determine if an individual is infected with HIV.) Meanwhile the couple will be learning more about each other. Details of history not recalled or consciously hidden at first may emerge, as may a drug or alcohol-dependence problem previously concealed, and—very important—

the six-month "slow" period provides opportunities for learning more about each other's trustworthiness.

Step 2

Swapping histories represents step 1 toward safer sex. (The process sounds tough already, doesn't it? It can be, but your health and possibly your life are on the line.)

Step 2 is equally necessary, because so many of us are unaware of sexually transmitted diseases unobtrusively residing within us. Step 2 involves each partner visiting a qualified physician or health facility for a thorough examination and laboratory testing for the presence of common sexually transmitted diseases, including HIV infection.

By law, the physician may report the results only to his or her patient, which means that if your partner is uncommunicative or failed to tell you the whole truth, you may really never get to know the results. Once again, there's a good reason for sticking to the highly inconvenient six months of the troublesome detailed routines involved in fending off sexually transmitted diseases.

Step 3

That brings us to step 3 of the approach toward safer sex, a process even more embarrassing than the open exchange of privacies in step 1.

Here we can learn something from prostitutes, those

specialists in casual sex who inspect their clients-to-be, concentrating on the penis, scrotum, and anal areas, and the adjacent thighs, buttocks, and lower abdomen. Some will look at the lips and mouth as well, checking for sores, discolorations, swellings, or other abnormalities indicative of disease. Many prostitutes will not allow purchasers of their services to kiss them on the mouth. The prostitute may ask the client to engage in a "short-arm" examination, a test borrowed from the armed services, in which the foreskin of the penis is pulled back, disclosing any abnormalities that may be hidden by it; the penis is pinched lightly at its base, the thumb on top and a finger underneath, and the fingers, squeezing gently, are slid along the length of the penis to its tip. Any fluid or discharge present in the urethra may appear at the opening in the tip of the penis.

Signs to look for include inflammation, sores, or other lesions (abnormal changes in the body tissue) that may indicate the presence of disease. If the man passes inspection, he should be asked to wash with soap and water, and, before being given full access to the pleasures anticipated, he must put on a condom.

A similar examination should be conducted on your partner each day that you have sexual intercourse. However ridiculous the process of mutual examination may seem (some might say it is suggestive of monkeys grooming each other), for safety's sake it must be done. The body may change from day to day, and fresh evidence of a developing infectious disease may appear. A basic rule of sexual safety is this: If there are signs or symptoms of a sexually transmitted disease, abstain from intercourse until a doctor declares sex is okay. If you sense something is wrong even though you cannot put your finger on anything specific, it would be safer for your emotional health to defer sexual interaction with a partner until you have no such reservations.

In the case of a heterosexual couple, the woman, Helen, would have the easier job. She could ask Michael whether he had noted any discharge from his penis or had suffered any pain in or near his genitals. His relevant parts being out in the open, she could readily manipulate and scan them, searching for lesions.

Helen, on the other hand, presents Michael with complex mysteries, with multiple folds requiring separation and good light for proper viewing, a deep, dark vagina that would require a gynecologist's expertise and equipment for truly adequate observation. In premenopausal women there is a normal discharge that even experts frequently find difficult to discern from an abnormal one. Normally, the vaginal fluid has a faint scent that most men find attractive. In this circumstance, the sense of smell may help, a malodorous discharge being more likely due to a disease process.

Michael and Helen are confronted with a need to establish the relative safety of each of their future couplings while operating with potentially flawed information. The histories they provided each other might not be totally dependable. Medical examinations and laboratory tests may, at times, provide misleading results. Their own amateur efforts at detecting disease in each other may fall short. There are uncertainties and hazards at every turn, and it's going to take time and trouble to keep these limited. Remember that each new partner means going through the same investigations and other routines—another incentive to limit the number of one's sexual partners. There will be many more steps in the pages that follow to help guide you through this precarious process.

Although most young people are probably not aware of it, the pleasures of sex are available to us for a lifetime if we retain our health. Many elderly people are sexually active. Senior citizens outside a long-standing, monogamous, faithful relationship should use the same safer sex measures their grandchildren or great-grandchildren do if they want to avoid sexually transmitted diseases. More and more of the elderly, many of them widows and widowers in their sixties, seventies, and eighties, are becoming involved with multiple sex partners and are subject to the risks that accompany such activities. HIV and other sexually transmitted diseases are now being reported more frequently in older age groups. Because of this none of the steps just detailed should be skipped simply because one believes he or she is too old for an STD.

6

Risks Come in All Sizes

Almost everything we do carries risks, including riding in a car, swimming in a pool, and, certainly, sexual intercourse.

In 1992, the New York State Department of Health charted the relative risks of catching HIV from an infected individual. Various types of unprotected sexual activity were examined.

The no-risk category included abstention; a faithful, monogamous relationship in which neither partner was infected; solo masturbation; massaging; touching, stroking, hugging; and social kissing (presumably with closed lips).

Deep kissing and mutual masturbation were rated as

activities having the lowest risk. Although saliva carries a low count of HIV, which correlates with the very low rate of infection through open mouth kissing, blood may have a high count of virus particles, and some people do have gums that bleed easily.

Cunnilingus and fellatio were also considered to be in the low-risk category.

The moderate-to-high-risk category for males included vaginal intercourse (the female infecting the male). But for females vaginal intercourse (the male infecting the female) was in the high-risk category.

Anal intercourse was rated as the activity with the highest risk because the rectum is easily torn, causing bleeding. In March 1989, *Consumer Reports* estimated that about one in 140 condoms broke during penile-vaginal intercourse. Considerably higher rates of condom breakage are likely in rectal intercourse, and with the bleeding so common in rectal intercourse the risk of HIV transmission goes up.

It is important to note that these risk categories apply only for HIV infection. Other sexually transmitted diseases have their own varied risks. For instance, social kissing was considered safe with respect to HIV infection, but anyone with an active "cold sore" on a lip due to herpes could transfer herpes to the recipient of that social kiss. Deep kissing was considered in the lowest-risk category for HIV infection, but it would be a high-risk activity if the kisser had active herpes in the mouth. Syphilis and a few other sexually transmitted diseases may also have sores and rashes with organisms in them transmissible on contact with an intact mucous membrane or with any area of skin with a break in its integrity. Condoms and other barrier methods provide protection for covered areas only.

From what has been said so far about the great value of condom use, it should be obvious that wise, sexually active individuals, female as well as male, should carry condoms with them at all times, so that they can be prepared for unplanned sexual intercourse.

Familiarity with the measures discussed throughout this book can further prepare you for unplanned sex, thereby reducing the risks of catching sexually transmitted diseases.

For those of us not content with abstention from sex, who are not in a long-standing monogamous relationship, who are not satisfied with solo sex, and who are unhappy with the limitations of safe, two-person sex, the next pages will carry instructions for minimizing the chances of falling victim to venereal disease.

Since every safety measure is fallible, high-risk activities are best avoided. If you do become involved in high-risk sex and your precautions fail, there are still things you can do to improve the odds and possibly reduce your risk of contracting a sexually transmitted disease. We'll come to these emergency rescue measures later.

Condoms are our foremost shields. They must be used every time because personal safety depends on them, which means every time a new relationship is begun and every time sex with a member of a high-risk category takes place. But remember that condoms, dental dams (a flat piece of very thin latex rubber), plastic wrap, rubber gloves, and so forth protect only the areas they cover. They give only incomplete protection against herpes, syphilis, and a number of other sexually transmitted diseases that may have lesions outside the locations covered effectively. Condoms serve a double purpose, that is, they protect well against most common venereal diseases and they are fairly effective in preventing pregnancy.

Unlubricated condoms, by reason of their neutral taste, are better for use in fellatio, but for other sexual purposes (i.e., vaginal or anal intercourse) condoms coated with a lubricant containing nonoxynol-9 are the choice. As has been mentioned, nonoxynol-9 is a spermicide that does a good job of killing microbes and viruses as well.

If a condom slips off—as it may if thrusting continues after ejaculation or if lubricating jelly was placed within the condom—or if the condom tears or leaks, the nonoxynol-9 is somewhat protective, but, to reinforce the defenses two applicatorsful of contraceptive jelly should be deposited in the vagina immediately after condom failure is recognized. That action may salvage the situation, preventing pregnancy and disease. In clinical practice this emergency measure seems to have been helpful, particularly with respect to gonorrheal and chlamydial* infections of the cervix. Whether nonoxy-

---

*Chlamydia are bacteria that can reproduce only within living cells. It is not required that the disease be reported to

nol-9 works as well in real-life as it does in test tubes in destroying HIV, the herpes virus, syphilis germs, and other organisms isn't known yet. The value of rectal administration of nonoxynol-9 in cases of condom failure in rectal intercourse is also unknown.

Barrier methods, that is, diaphragms and cervical caps, back up the efficacy of condom use as a contraceptive and, to some extent, as a disease preventive.

An intrauterine device (IUD), although very effective in preventing pregnancy, may make infection of the uterus and fallopian tubes more likely by such bacteria as chlamydia, gonorrhea, streptococcus, staphylococcus, and coli. Because of this, some physicians advise those of their patients who are not in a long-standing, faithful, monogamous relationship to discontinue use of the IUD in favor of a different method of birth control.

Use of sufficient lubricant within the vagina may reduce the approximately one in one hundred breakage rate of condoms. Similarly, lubricating the anal region liberally for anal intercourse may lessen that breakage rate from between one in four and ten to a less worrisome level.

---

health authorities, but it is one of the most common of the sexually transmitted diseases (STDs) in the United States. Chlamydia come in different strains, each strain often producing very different illnesses. Some will produce eye diseases, others lymphogranuloma venereum (discussed later), but most commonly some cause infection of the urogenital tract in men and women. Chlamydia will be discussed in further detail later.

As suggested before, a condom should be used for at least the first six months of a new relationship, because it may take that long for a newly acquired infection to register a positive test. Both partners should be tested for HIV at six months into their relationship to catch virtually all the positive tests, although testing at three months detects most of the positives.

This seems like a good place to emphasize the obvious. Unless for some reason that would escape most of us you are looking forward to a tragic life with more than its share of anxiety, pain, frustration, and rage against fate, you should not, ever, skip any of the safety precautions we're considering here. On the occasion when you might be very tired, or a little drunk or high, or just plain lazy, and you don't want to bother going to the bathroom for your supplies, and you tell yourself, "The odds of anything happening are so small, just this once I'm going to skip it!" remember that you are wrong! Don't play Russian roulette with your future. That trifling unprotected risk can be responsible for an unwanted pregnancy and it may start an illness that could kill you. In short, try not to do anything foolish, and don't omit any of the steps provided here to add to your safety and peace of mind.

The assorted advisories that follow are intended to shelter you, as much as possible, from the heavy weather in the current sex scene. Don't be surprised at encountering repetition along the way, it helps important lessons stick in one's memory.

Tips for Reducing Risks

The first bit of street smarts, which has already been mentioned, might almost fit into a wordy fortune cookie: Appearance of glowing good health is no guarantee of freedom from sexually transmitted diseases. The rigorous steps for establishing the suitability of a sex partner must never be ignored or overlooked.

You can improve your chances of remaining healthy by pruning your potential sex partners to exclude high-risk individuals. You would be well advised not to have sex with anyone who falls into one or more of the following groups:

- those who have themselves tested positive for HIV or have had a lover test positive for HIV;
- those who have had numerous sex partners;
- those who have used drugs hypodermically or have had sex with someone who has used drugs hypodermically;
- those who have adventured sexually abroad, particularly in tropical and semitropical regions; and
- those who will not employ the protective measures you feel are necessary to protect your physical and mental health.

As already mentioned, the fewer your sex partners, the less likely you are to become infected with a sexually transmitted disease.

Under the influence of alcohol or drugs, we are all

capable of acting irresponsibly. If you are serious about remaining as safe as possible from venereal diseases, you have to stick to your entire protection regimen, which means you should not drink or do drugs.

It's important to recognize the early patterns of illness found in those with sexually transmitted diseases, because rapid medical consultation will help to minimize the damage done to the body. Brief descriptions of each of the sexually transmitted diseases are given in a later section of this book. In general one should look for sores in or near the genital area or rashes not previously present, vaginal or penile discharges that are new or increased, burning on urination, itching in the genital or anal regions, warts in the anogenital regions, pain in the lower abdomen or groin, and swellings.

If the symptoms or signs of a sexually transmitted disease clear up spontaneously after days or weeks, don't be fooled into thinking: "Good! That took care of itself!" Some of the venereal diseases have a limited acute phase; then the germs go into hiding places in the body, with all sorts of nasty consequences possible (for example, sterility or damage to the cardiovascular system, central nervous system, or bones). Make it your policy to see your doctor early in the development of abnormalities. Also, you should be aware that development of immunity to a sexually transmitted disease is rare. Unlike the chicken pox and some other childhood diseases, most sexually transmitted diseases can be caught repeatedly.

Vaginal soreness or irritation of the penis during sexual intercourse is a signal to discontinue the sexual activity. These symptoms may indicate the presence of tiny abrasions that may readily become infected. If the symptoms persist, or if there is persistent pain on intercourse, a doctor should be consulted.

As has been stated previously, if you know you have a sexually transmitted disease, or if there is anything to suggest that you or your partner might have one, discontinue sexual relations immediately. See your doctor as soon as possible, follow all instructions as closely as you can, and do not resume sexual relations until your doctor says it's all right to do so. Even in a case as trivial as pubic lice which you have diagnosed yourself, you should probably still see your doctor. When you picked up the lice you might also have picked up another sexually transmitted disease.

If you are sexually active and not in a long-standing, faithful relationship, it's worthwhile to see your physician annually for an examination and for laboratory testing for syphilis, gonorrhea, chlamydia, and other sexually transmitted diseases. HIV testing should also certainly be done, although you may wish to do this somewhere other than your doctor's office for reasons of privacy (this will be discussed in more detail in the section on HIV). An annual checkup is advised because, as we have said, you may have acquired a sexually transmitted disease but, as often happens, it has not demonstrated enough symptoms to make you aware of its existence. For many of the venereal infections, the lack of symptoms is more common among women than men, but in the case of HIV, men and women equally may carry the virus infections for ten years or more without any obvious lesions.

Unless a condom is used, fellatio may result in gonorrhea, syphilis, genital herpes, chlamydia, warts, hepatitis, or maybe HIV. Infection by some of these diseases becomes even more likely if ejaculation into the mouth occurs. An infected woman receiving cunnilingus may transmit genital warts, genital herpes, syphilis, hepatitis, gonorrhea, chlamydia, and maybe HIV to her partner if no rubber dam or plastic barrier is used. Rinsing the mouth immediately after unprotected cunnilingus or fellatio may lower the risk of infection, but oral sex of any kind should be avoided if there are any inflammations about the mouth or the genital area.

Mutual masturbation, stimulating each other manually, is reasonably safe if a partner's body fluids do not get in or on the other's body. Barrier methods should be used, including rubber gloves, the kind medical personnel wear, to protect the hands.

Hands are active participants in most love-making and should be washed as often as possible. Rubber gloves should be worn when fingers are going to enter the vagina or rectum, as ungloved hands may pick up sexually transmitted diseases through tiny cuts or abrasions.

After contact with the anus by hand, mouth, or penis without the barrier protection of a condom, glove, dental dam, or plastic wrap, any body parts directly involved must be thoroughly washed with soap and water. If barrier methods have been used, a fresh condom, glove, or whatever, must be used before the vulva and vagina are approached.

Bathing before a sexual encounter is desirable for most people. But for those with many sexual partners bathing as soon as feasible after sex is necessary to increase the odds of being safe from infection. Any part of the body wetted by a partner's body fluids should be washed thoroughly with soap and water. This means the lather should be allowed to remain on the skin for at least fifteen seconds before rinsing to enhance its germ-killing power. Although the intact skin is a tough, protective shield against most infections, it takes only tiny cuts or abrasions to allow infectious agents through.

Having said that, it is now easy to see that you should avoid any sexual activity that may cause bleeding. The human immunodeficiency virus and other venereal infections are readily transmitted by blood and will easily pass through any cut or abrasion. Avoid sharing razors, toothbrushes, douching or enema equipment, sex toys, or anything that might have been contaminated by blood. If you have any doubt as to the sterilization of the instruments used, don't get any tattoos, shaves by a barber, acupuncture, or hypodermic injections.

If you are going to have surgery, speak to your surgeon about arranging to donate your own blood ahead of time so it is available should you require a transfusion during or after the operation. Currently, the blood supply in the United States is very safe, and blood contaminated with HIV or anything else rarely slips by, but your own blood would be safest of all.*

In some countries outside the United States, however, the standards governing the purity of the blood supply are not as strict, and therefore it would be a good idea to try to avoid transfusions abroad. (Of course, not many people plan to spend their vacations abroad in the hospital receiving transfusions, but since blood is such a well-known carrier of infectious organisms, this caveat should not be disregarded.)

It is wise to wash areas of skin exposed to the blood or body fluids of an HIV-infected individual with soap and water, or with 3 percent hydrogen peroxide (the kind used for rinsing cuts), or with a dilute solution of household bleach (one part bleach to nine parts water), or povidone iodine solution, or 70 percent rubbing alcohol to help prevent a new HIV infection. (Alcohol is not advised for use on sensitive parts, such as the vulva or penis since it can dry and irritate sensitive tissues and mucous membranes.) The same methods should considerably lessen the menace of skin contact with the infected fluids, blood, or lesions of the other venereal diseases.

If they are able to tolerate such treatment, sex toys (dildos, battery-operated vibrators, etc.) can be cleaned

---

*The risk of HIV from a transfusion of a single unit of blood is 1:250,000; for Hepatitis B it is 1:200,000; for Hepatitis C it is 1:3,300. Statistics taken from L. Tierney et al., eds., *Current Medical Diagnosis and Treatment* (Stamford, Conn.: Appleton and Lange, 1997).

by a hot water and soap wash, followed by immersion for fifteen minutes in a solution of household bleach (one part bleach to nine parts water) and then a tap water rinse.

In spite of their bad reputation in the public's eye, toilet seats very rarely act as agents for the transfer of sexually transmitted diseases. However, if it makes you feel safer, cover public toilet seats with toilet paper or the sanitary paper cover some restrooms provide, first having made sure the seat is dry.

One additional precaution is easy to take. As soon as it is convenient after a sexual encounter, urinate. Germs that may have found their way into the urethra may be washed away by the stream of urine prior to establishing an infection. (A number of authorities recommend this action, but we have no firm evidence that it accomplishes what we hope.)

The term "safer sex" usually refers to reducing the chances of acquiring a sexually transmitted disease, but it also includes avoidance of pregnancy when pregnancy is not a goal. Although the birth control pill is an effective contraceptive, many women seem unaware that it is designed strictly for that purpose: to prevent pregnancy from occurring. They seem to feel that while they are taking the pill they are protected from all potentially adverse effects of engaging in intercourse. Birth control pills are not prophylactics; they were not designed to prevent venereal diseases. To avoid acquiring a sexually transmitted disease while simultaneously preventing pregnancy, a birth control method other than the pill must be used. Some popular, successful options include condoms, diaphragms, and other barrier methods, especially when used in conjunction with contraceptive jellies or foams containing an effective spermicide like nonoxynol-9.

The depth of emotional attachment and sense of commitment differ among sexual partners, but responsible behavior means that in all your dealings with sexual partners you will try in your speech and actions to produce as much joy for both of you as you can and cause as little shame, humiliation, guilt, or other negative feelings as possible. Safer sex requires the involvement of all participants. Anyone who has been informed that he or she has a sexually transmitted disease has an obligation to tell all of his or her sexual partners, tactfully and sensitively, so that they can seek prompt medical attention.

We live in a fast-moving era, with scientists pouring out new findings, some of which may apply to the avoidance and treatment of sexually transmitted diseases. It is wise to keep sampling the media for medical developments that may affect you directly and that you may wish to discuss with your doctor.

7

Presenting: Sexually Transmitted Diseases

Having gone through the many burdensome steps necessary to make free-ranging sex safer, the sexual lifestyles that do not require those many encumbrances may now appear more inviting: At one end of the spectrum is the option of a faithful, disease-free, monogamous relationship; at the other, the shunning of any form of direct sexual expression; and, somewhere in between, solo sexual practices (masturbation) and risk-free activities such as dancing and hugging. But please defer any lifestyle decisions until you've read the rest of this book.

Now you are about to come face-to-face with the enemy's armed forces, the individual sexually trans-

mitted diseases (STDs), roughly thirty in all.* My aim is
not to appall but to inform, to let you know what to
watch for if you are unlucky enough, or careless enough,
to contract one or more of these unlovely souvenirs of
what may have been a very lovely and passionate sexual
encounter. I also hope to teach you to recognize what it
is you're finding when you spot lesions on a partner.

These STDs are organized so that the lesser-known,
less common ones are presented first. Pronunciation
keys for those which may be unfamiliar to readers are
included as footnotes. Diseases with similar symptoms
are grouped together in chapters, but the best-known,
most common STDs, such as AIDS and herpes, have
individual chapters devoted to them.

Only enough detail to serve your needs is provided
about each. It's not possible to list all the possible ways
in which an STD may present itself, but for each I have
included there will be early, fairly characteristic symptoms and signs to enable you to recognize conditions
that can endanger you or your partner.

Most of the time I will not specify the names of
antibiotics or other agents of treatment. In the medical
world changes in the management of an illness may
occur quite rapidly, and what is written today may well
become outdated tomorrow. Your doctor stays on top of
current developments and is your best source for up-to-
date treatment information.

---

*The number of STDs differs from text to text, depending
on the criteria used to include this or that disease.

Now it's time to see just what it is you'll be guarding against.

Balanoposthitis*

Although not strictly a sexually transmitted disease, balanoposthitis is included in this listing because so many of the sexually transmitted diseases may participate in causing this condition, which most people—I'm sure—have never heard of. Balanoposthitis is the inflammation of the head of the penis or clitoris and the overlying prepuce. The term is derived from balanitis, an inflammation of the head (glans) of the penis or clitoris, and posthitis, an inflammation of the foreskin (prepuce). In males who have been circumcised and have had the entire foreskin removed there can be no posthitis.

The inflammation often develops two or three days after sexual intercourse, but it may occur without any history of sexual contact. It may also occur during a bout of gonorrhea, herpes simplex, trichomoniasis, candidiasis, or syphilis (each of which will be discussed later), or during a variety of noninfectious skin disorders. A tight foreskin, difficult or impossible to retract, is a predisposing factor, as in men with diabetes mellitus ("sugar diabetes").

Balanoposthitis frequently causes a discharge from under the foreskin, ulcerations of the foreskin and the

---

*(bal'-an-o-pos-thigh'-tis)

glans, soreness and redness of the areas involved, and enlargement and tenderness of the lymph nodes in the groin.

Laboratory tests that the physician might order would include smears and cultures of the discharge, investigations for sexually transmitted diseases that might be associated with the inflammation, tests of the urine and blood for sugar to determine if diabetes mellitus is present, and blood tests for syphilis and any other conditions the circumstances call for.

If no specific cause of the inflammation is found, a salt solution is used to rinse the site several times a day. If ordinary bacteria appear to have caused a secondary infection, the drugs used to fight that infection should be chosen carefully so that any early symptoms of syphilis will not be masked. If a tight foreskin is a contributing factor, when the acute phase of the inflammation has cleared, circumcision should be considered, to prevent irritating collections of smegma from forming and to lessen chances of a balanitis recurring. The transitory pain of adult circumcision, which is easily controlled with oral pain medication, is far preferable to the dangers associated with a tight foreskin, one of which is cancer of the penis.

Reiter's Syndrome

Reiter's syndrome is not a sexually transmitted disease, but it is a disease that may be brought on by sex. A defined cause has not yet been determined but there appear to be two major precipitating events: an intestinal infection with one of several kinds of bacteria, such as Salmonella; and a urinary tract infection or infection of the cervix, most often a chlamydia infection. Particularly in children and the elderly, and equally in male and female, it seems frequently to follow an intestinal infection. When Reiter's occurs as a consequence of sexual intercourse, it strikes mostly men between the ages of twenty and forty. Women seem to be less likely than men to get Reiter's syndrome after sex, but it may be that their illness is simply milder and therefore harder to recognize.

There are four major components to Reiter's syndrome, but they usually do not appear simultaneously; sometimes they appear weeks apart: an eye inflammation, arthritis of a number of joints, inflammation of the genito-urinary tract, and lesions of the mucous membranes and skin.

In sexually transmitted diseases, the organism responsible can usually be found in the patient's body, and tests will disclose its presence. In Reiter's no such organism has ever been isolated from the parts exhibiting inflammation, and there is no test that establishes the diagnosis.

Instead, the diagnosis is based on the clinical picture of the arthritis pattern (involvement mostly of weight-bearing joints, such as knees and ankles and of the lower back and spine), eye inflammations, skin and mucous membrane rashes, and the presence at some stage of the illness of urethritis (inflammation of the urethra) or cervicitis (inflammation of the cervix).

There is another important difference from the standard sexually transmitted diseases: Reiter's syndrome cannot be transferred to anyone else by sexual contact with the patient.

A theoretical explanation of what goes on in Reiter's is that certain sexually transmitted organisms and organisms that cause dysentery share chemical resemblances with parts of the body. Because of this the immune mechanisms organized to attack the invaders also attack the tissues in the eyes, the urethra, a small number of joints, and the skin and mucous membranes bearing chemical similarities to the organisms.

One or two weeks after sexual intercourse or an episode of dysentery, the Reiter's syndrome patient will develop, at different times, a low fever; inflammation of the mucous membranes of the eyes; arthritis of some joints, mostly in the lower extremities and back; and urethritis or cervicitis. Various eruptions may appear on the skin and mucous membranes. The initial attack is usually self-limited (i.e., one that clears up without any treatment other than what the body itself provides), but the arthritis may persist for a few years, and, in about one in five of the patients, lasting joint damage may occur. There may be recurrences, some of which may follow sexual contacts

Reiter's syndrome, fortunately, is not a common condition. It occurs in only 2 percent of males with nongonorrheal urethritis (inflammation of the urethra caused by something other than gonorrhea), and in 2 to 3 percent of patients with dysentery due to certain bacteria.

Whether antibiotics have any value in treating this syndrome is controversial. Symptoms are treated with appropriate medications.

8

"Mostly Female" Troubles

Bacterial Vaginosis*

The fact that medicine is an inexact science is well exemplified by bacterial vaginosis (also known as Haemophilus vaginalis vaginitis, or, by a newer name, as Gardnerella vaginalis vaginitis), because the cause of the disease is controversial. So is the mode of transmission, sexual according to some texts, nonsexual according to others.

Apparently upsetting the balanced environment of the vagina and disturbing the organisms at home there

---

*(bak-tee'-ree-àl vaj'-i-no-sàs)

may bring on an episode of bacterial vaginosis. Among factors altering the balance may be such agents as antibiotics, tampons, certain vaginal hygiene products, and some commercial lubricants.

Vaginosis is a very common condition that may appear as a vaginal discharge with an unpleasant or fishy odor, or it may cause so little alteration that some women live with it for months or years assuming that the minor change is normal. In some women vulval soreness may occur, but this is uncommon.

Supporting the belief that vaginosis is transmitted sexually is the finding that women who are sexually active have Gardnerella in the vagina more often than women who are sexually inexperienced. Also Gardner in 1955 and Pheifer in 1978 found *Gardnerella vaginalis* in the urethras of 78 percent and 80 percent respectively of the male sex partners of women with bacterial vaginosis, but not in the urethras of men whose partners did not have bacterial vaginosis. Then B. Piol et al. in 1984 found that the Gardnerella subtypes from women with bacterial vaginosis were the same subtypes that were isolated from their male partners more often than chance alone would explain, suggesting that sexual intercourse supplied a reasonable explanation.*

Previously it was believed that the predominantly causative organism for bacterial vaginosis was *Gardnerella vaginalis*, but now it seems that other organisms

---

*See King K. Holmes, et al., eds., *Sexually Transmitted Diseases* (New York: McGraw-Hill, 1990).

may act in concert with that particular bacterium. However, we don't know for sure. What we do know is that many young women who have not had any sexual exposure do get bacterial vaginosis nonsexually.

A combination of findings helps to establish the diagnosis. On examination there is usually a thin gray or white adherent vaginal discharge, which, when tested with litmus paper, is found to be less acid than normal. Further tests are done to verify the diagnosis of bacterial vaginosis. For example, the "whiff test" may be performed: a drop of a 10 percent solution of potassium hydroxide is added to a drop of vaginal fluid. If bacterial vaginosis is present, a strong, fishy odor is released. (Appropriately, this is known as a "whiff" test.) A further bit of detective work involves examining a stained smear of vaginal fluid microscopically (staining a slide containing biological material will highlight certain features for study under a microscope). If vaginosis is present, the edges of the flat, superficial cells that line the vaginal surface will be dotted with bacteria. Microscopic examination will also demonstrate that lactobacilli bacteria, plentiful in a normal vagina, are scant or absent.

Men who have sex with women suffering from vaginosis rarely develop symptoms, and they rarely receive treatment.

Unfortunately the standard antibiotics are not very effective in treating bacterial vaginosis. The chemotherapeutic agent most used in trichomoniasis, a disease which will be discussed next, is usually the agent of choice for bacterial vaginosis. A group of gynecologists has found that eight out of ten women who have been successfully treated will get bacterial vaginosis again within nine months, and providing treatment to male sexual partners does not affect the recurrence rate.

As with all such conditions, your doctor's instructions should be followed as closely as possible.

Trichomoniasis*

An actively swimming microscopic, one-celled animal, *Trichomonas vaginalis*, can cause a foul discharge that may go on for years if not treated. No matter if she has just bathed, no matter how well dressed she is or how beautifully groomed, awareness of this malodorous discharge may tend to make a woman feel unclean and maybe unlovable, seriously damaging her self-image.

Worldwide, trichomoniasis is one of the most common sexually transmitted diseases, but it is not a dangerous illness in relation to other STDs. The organism that causes trichomoniasis attaches itself only to parts of the genito-urinary lining of women and men, where it may produce no symptoms at all and does little lasting harm.

After an incubation period of four to twenty days, women may experience a vaginal discharge and inflammation, with associated redness of the vulva, irritation or itching, uncomfortable urination, painful intercourse,

---

*(trik'-o-mo-neye'-à-sis)

and, less commonly, discomfort of the lower abdomen. Most men, however, have no symptoms. Other men may suffer from a urethritis caused by trichomonads, the parasitic, single-celled organisms that cause trichomoniasis, with distress on voiding and a discharge from the penis. The urinary bladder and the prostate gland may also be infected. Most men seek medical attention because they are sexual partners of women who have been diagnosed with trichomoniasis. A majority of men, even if untreated, seem to rid themselves of the trichomonads in weeks, unlike women, who must obtain medical intervention to be cured.

For years the treatment of choice has been metronidazole, a chemotherapeutic agent. It is important that sexual partners be treated simultaneously so that the untreated partner does not cause reinfection of the partner receiving treatment and sex should be avoided until cure is established in both partners.

Cystitis*

Cystitis, a urinary bladder infection that, on occasion, follows soon after sexual intercourse, is usually caused by germs that normally live in the patient's colon, and not by bacteria responsible for the sexually transmitted diseases. The disease occurs mostly in females and is caused by the bacteria migrating up the urethra (which,

---

*(sis-tie'-tis)

you will recall, is considerably shorter in females than in males) and into the urinary bladder. The cystitis patient may have such uncomfortable symptoms as frequency of urination, an urgent sense of needing to urinate even after the bladder has just been emptied, burning or pain on urination, and bloody urine.

In rear-entry vaginal intercourse—the male facing his partner's back—the penis striking against the front wall of the vagina is more likely to bring on a cystitis than in other coital positions, because the urethra and bladder lie just beyond that wall.

The most frequent bacterial agent in cystitis, *Escherichia coli*, is the predominant organism in the normal bowel movement. Wiping from back to front after a bowel movement, as some women do, introduces foreign germs to the vulva and the urethral opening, allowing them easier access to the bladder. This unhygienic wiping practice may also—in theory, at least—make unprotected cunnilingus as risky as putting the mouth and tongue to the anus. Early in life, girls should be taught to wipe only from vulva to anus (front to rear) and never from anus to vulva.

Urinating right after intercourse may serve to wash away some of the bacteria from the urethral opening, but it is not enough to bring peace of mind to some women, who may choose to take a hurried douche.

If symptoms suggestive of acute cystitis become more than occasional brief events, you should see your physician. If you must visit your physician on a regular basis for the same symptoms, he or she may allow you to treat yourself with a prescription drug. If you have as many as three episodes a year, your physician may want to put you on daily doses (or some other dosage schedule) of antibiotics and/or chemotherapeutic agents, because inadequately treated cystitis may lead to kidney damage.

Candidiasis* ("Yeast Infection")

A maddening itch is the primary symptom that many women associate with candidiasis, also known as moniliasis or monilia, a yeast infection of the mucous membranes. This infection may strike the vagina, rectum, and mouth, or the skin and other parts of the body.

Candida albicans, the organism most commonly associated with candidiasis, causes about one in five cases of vaginitis. *Candida* is a normal resident of the vagina, a well-behaved tenant under ordinary circumstances, but the number of yeast cells will proliferate, causing a disease state, if the environmental balance in the vagina is disturbed. Common predisposing factors include hormonal changes produced by pregnancy or by contraceptive pills, the use of broad-spectrum antibiotics, and changes in blood-sugar levels such as those caused by diabetes mellitus.

The major signs and symptoms are a curdy, white vaginal discharge, which may be scant, redness of the

---

*(can-di-dyé-a-sis)

vulva and vagina, itching, painful voiding, and painful intercourse.

Sexual intercourse may transfer the yeast to the male, and about 10 percent of the male partners will develop inflammation of the penis and foreskin and experience painful urination.

The diagnosis of candidiasis is usually made after microscopically examining stained smears from the vagina or penis, but the use of tissue cultures increases positive diagnoses by about 25 percent.

Local treatment with the antifungal agents now available, over the counter as well as by prescription, will usually clear up the condition, but recurrences are common. Many women who become all too familiar with the nature of their affliction due to recurrent attacks will treat themselves. Control of predisposing conditions (such as the use of contraceptive pills, or wearing tight jeans or nylon underpants) is necessary if recurrences are to be reduced.

Sexual intercourse may be resumed when the physician has determined that all signs and symptoms of candidiasis are gone.

9

The Itch You Just Can't Scratch

Tinea Cruris*

Tinea cruris, a type of ringworm commonly known as jock itch, is a common infection of the skin of the upper portion of the inner thighs and adjacent groin, and, occasionally, of the scrotum and external labia and the skin between the buttocks caused by various fungi, including that which we call ringworm. The infection flourishes in conditions of warmth, moisture, and the friction caused by skin rubbing against skin. When the upper inner thighs have the right conditions of moisture, heat, and superficial

---

*(tin'-ee-à croo'-ris)

abrasions, specialized fungi, usually present on the skin, will start an infection of the outer layers of the skin. Jock itch is only mildly contagious, but thereby gains its right to be listed as a sexually transmitted disease, because long-standing partners may catch it. Tinea cruris used to be almost entirely a male disorder, but, in recent years, has gone female as well, since women have taken to wearing snug-fitting underwear and slacks that interfere with the evaporation of moisture from the pelvic area.

Jock itch appears as tan, grayish, or reddish sharply defined scaly patches, sometimes with tiny bumps along the edges. In mild cases there may be little or no itching. Chronic itching, however, may lead to chronic scratching, resulting in the thickening of the skin, sometimes with a superimposed bacterial infection (i.e., one infection on top of a previous one).

Topical antifungal agents are available, as are others that can be taken by mouth. In either regimen improvement is slow and treatment lengthy. Relapse is common.

Wearing loose-fitting cotton underwear, and, for women, skirts instead of slacks, would help conditions by improving ventilation, as would avoiding blue jeans and other tightly knit trousers.

Scabies*

Sarcoptes scabiei, the itch mite, which belongs to the same class of eight-legged bugs as spiders and ticks, is a tiny

---

*(skay'-beez)

parasite barely visible to the naked eye. It lives in bur-
rows in the outer layer of the skin which may be seen as
fine wavy lines. The mites deposit eggs in these little
tunnels and the larvae hatch in a few days

Symptoms of infestation first occur three or four
weeks after its start. It it is believed that an allergic reac-
tion to the mites, their saliva, or their excretory products
leads to the severe itching which is more intense at
night, when the warmth of bed covers exacerbates the
itching. This itching provokes vigorous scratching that
may lead to bacterial skin infections.

The mites are spread by skin-to-skin contact, as will
occur in sexual relations, or by using infected bedding or
towels. Mites that are shed from the body die very
quickly.

A scabies infection frequently starts in the genital
region (characteristic red bumps may appear on the
head and shaft of the penis) but soon spreads to the
webs of the fingers, the armpits, hands, wrists, ankles,
elbows, buttocks, and breasts (in females). The scalp and
face of an adult are usually not involved.

Diagnosis is made by identifying the mites or their
eggs during the microscopic examination of material
scraped from one of the tiny tunnels.

Treatment from the neck down with chemicals that
kill the mites and their eggs usually results in cure, but
itching goes on for another few weeks.

Because symptoms take nearly a month to develop,
sexual partners should be treated even if no indications
of scabies are found.

Pubic Lice

Pthirus pubis, the pubic louse, is a flat wingless insect with tiny legs that resembles a freckle. It lives on blood it sucks through the skin. It favors the anogenital region and lays its eggs (nits) on the hairs there, close to the skin. In hairy individuals, pubic lice may be found as far away from the genital region as the eyebrows. The chief symptom is itching.

Toilet seats, which are notorious in the public mind as the source of much disease, are rarely responsible for causing any of the sexually transmitted diseases, but they may occasionally be responsible for a case of pubic lice. The nit-bearing hairs shed by an infected person may be left on the public toilet seat, only to become tangled in the genital hairs of the next person to sit down. Shortly thereafter, an embarrassing, annoying itch would proclaim that pubic lice had taken up residence.

To prevent transmission through this medium, either avoid sitting on the toilet seat, or, after making sure the seat is dry, cover it with toilet tissue or with the special paper covers provided in some public restrooms before sitting. Sexual transmission is the most common medium, but shared clothing or bedding may also play a role in passing lice along.

Diagnosis is made by finding adult lice, which may be few in number, or their nits.

Cure in over 90 percent of cases follows just one application of a lotion containing a chemical toxic to lice and nits. After one week, if any lice are found, retreatment is called for.

Sexual partners should be checked by a physician, not only for lice, but also for other sexually transmitted diseases that might have been transferred at the same time.

Enterobiasis*

The chief symptom of enterobiasis (pinworm infestation) is itching of the anal region, particularly during the night, when it may be severe enough to disrupt sleep. The most prominent victims of invasion by *Enterobius vermicularis* are young children who do a poor job of washing their hands. Having soiled their hands with stool after having had a bowel movement, children are liable to contaminate almost anything and everything in their environment: food, clothing, furniture, bedding, toys, and so on. Even the dust in the daycare center, classroom, or home may have pinworm eggs in it.

Because the eggs in the environment remain viable for up to two weeks, if a child in the family has pinworms, adults who are hasty, or careless, in hand washing before eating will ingest the eggs and develop worms. Unprotected oral-anal sex can lead to sexual transmission of the disease. It takes about three to four weeks for a mature egg-laying female to develop from a swallowed egg.

The itching during the night results from the female

*(en'-tàr-o-beye'-à-sis)

pinworm coming out of the anus to lay her eggs. The itch provokes scratching, which leads to abrasions, which may in turn lead to infections of the skin of the anal region and sometimes to inflammation of the vulva and vagina. Many of those who have pinworms present no symptoms. Other symptoms are involuntary loss of urine, restlessness, and irritability, affecting children mostly. Some individuals remain asymptomatic, sleeping through the nocturnal wanderings of the egg-laying worms.

The diagnosis is usually made in a most interesting way. The first thing in the morning a strip of transparent plastic tape is applied, sticky-side down, against the skin around the anus. It is immediately removed and applied sticky-side down onto a glass slide and scanned through a microscope. The *Enterobius eggs,* if they are present, are readily identified. Occasionally live worms may be seen on the stool in the toilet bowl, though this is a less frequent method of diagnosis.

Chemotherapeutic agents usually cure the infestation. Careful hand-washing before eating may prevent a recurrence. The use of plastic wrap or a rubber dental dam in all oral-anal sex is certainly recommended.

10

Viral Hepatitis

Most of us recognize the term "jaundice," a condition in which the skin and the white of the eyes turn yellow. The yellow fever virus may dye us yellow, as may the measles virus, herpes simplex, and assorted other viruses, drugs, toxic agents, tumors, and so on.

The focus here, however, will be the mixed group of viruses known for their attack on the liver, sometimes producing an illness so mild as to go unnoticed or, rarely, so severe as to kill. Each of these liver inflammations is known as a viral hepatitis, and scientists have identified five of the culprits, labeling them hepatitis A, B, C, D, and E. As of 1997 F and G have also been identified, but as yet little is known about them. Hepatitis A

and B are known to be sexually transmitted at times, and
it appears highly possible that the others are as well.

All five varieties of hepatitis initiate illness in the
same pattern, causing malaise, loss of appetite, nausea,
vomiting, and sometimes fever. Other milder, nonspecific symptoms, such as muscle ache, headache, and
joint pain, may also be evident. These symptoms may
indicate any number of illnesses, and it is not until some
days after infection has occurred that viral hepatitis
announces itself. Symptoms that would indicate the
presence of hepatitis include the urine getting darker
and the stool lighter a few days before yellowness of the
eyes and skin first appears. Smokers may experience an
aversion to smoking. An ache may develop in the upper
right portion of the abdomen and a physician may be
able to palpate an enlarged liver, with the patient com-
plaining of tenderness there. Acute viral hepatitis also
frequently leads to a loss of sexual desire.

Blood samples gathered to assess liver function and
state-of-the-art studies of immune substances produced
by the patient are necessary for the diagnosis of viral
hepatitis to be made and to determine which specific
virus is responsible.

The treatment of acute viral hepatitis is largely based
on treating the symptoms, for we have no cure. Abstinence from sexual activity during acute illness is recommended. Because hepatitis can be transmitted through
casual contact, sexual partners, household, and other
close contacts of the patient should be seen by a physician as soon as practical. Caught early enough, it may be

be possible to prevent illness in those already or soon to be infected.

The hepatitis viruses, for all their similarities in early clinical behavior, differ considerably in certain respects. Each virus, A, B, C, D, and E, will be discussed one at a time for an analysis of their dissimilarities.

Hepatitis A

Hepatitis A virus (HAV) infection is seldom serious; in fact, many infected individuals never become aware of any discomfort, although they are capable of spreading the infection, largely by way of the virus in their stools.

Infection comes from eating raw or inadequately cooked shellfish taken from waters contaminated by bowel movements containing HAV, or by drinking water from a similarly contaminated source. Infected food handlers who fail to wash their hands properly (as with soap and water for at least fifteen seconds) after a bowel movement can also spread the disease. Oral-anal contact and fellatio on a penis that has acquired HAV through contact with the anal region both represent sexually transmitted routes. Unlike most other sexually transmitted diseases, which can be caught over and over again, an established HAV infection results in a lifetime immunity.

It takes ten to fifty days for symptoms to appear in those who do get sick, but the virus is in their body fluids and can infect others before any symptoms develop. Once jaundice is established, the patient usually starts feeling better.

The patient remains contagious until about a week after jaundice appears. Therefore, once the diagnosis is made, sexual partners and household and other close contacts are usually given gamma globulin injections. If given within two weeks of exposure to the HAV, gamma globulin* will prevent the development of clinical illness 80 to 90 percent of the time. Convalescence and full recovery usually take up to several months, although clinical or biochemical relapses may extend the recovery period as long as a year.

HAV infection has no chronic carrier state and there are no long-term consequences to the illness. In the elderly, a severe HAV infection will occasionally result in death (the mortality rate is 0.2 percent).

Because HAV infection is quite prevalent, it is worth discussing the advisability of prophylactic injections of gamma globulin with your physician if you will be traveling abroad. The usual dose is protective for about six weeks, but a larger dose will work for five or six months.

---

*Gamma globulin is the fraction of whole blood, pooled from about two hundred apparently normal individuals, that contains the specific immune substances that these individuals have generated during their lifetime exposures to viruses and other infections. Since hepatitis A is so prevalent, some of these immune substances are almost certain to be against hepatitis A virus.

Hepatitis B

The hepatitis B virus (HBV) infection is much like HAV infection, but there are important differences. For example, hepatitis B may be more gradual in onset than A. Like A, there may be individuals infected with HBV who never get sick, but, unlike A, 5 to 10 percent will become chronic carriers of the virus. Some will have a smoldering case of hepatitis for years, and of these, some cases will clear up spontaneously. But about 40 percent of chronic hepatitis patients will develop cirrhosis of the liver and a smaller number may also contract liver cell cancer, both frequently fatal.

Worldwide, most HBV infections occur in the first few years of life, during pregnancy or delivery, when the mother is a carrier, or by as yet unknown channels, such as through contact with infected family members or other individuals. In the United States, however, HBV is often sexually transmitted. Male homosexuals with multiple sex partners are particularly at risk, although heterosexual transmission has increased recently.

HBV is probably present in all the body fluids of an infected person, but in some fluids is so sparsely present, as in tears or breast milk, as not to have demonstrated infectiousness. Stools are not a factor in the spread of HBV as they are with HAV.

Blood and other body fluids, such as semen, vaginal secretions, and saliva, are vehicles for sexual spread, whereas nonsexual spread frequently occurs by injection. Examples of this type of transmission would include drug addicts sharing unclean equipment; or health-care workers such as physicians, dentists, nurses, and laboratory technicians being accidentally wounded by contaminated instruments; or the exposure of lacerated or abraded skin areas to infectious body fluids.

The incubation period for HBV may be anywhere from six weeks to six months. HBV may be transmissible from one to six weeks before there are any signs or symptoms of illness.

Ordinary gamma globulin may not be effective in aborting illness, even given as early as one to two days after exposure to HBV, but hepatitis B immune globulin is very effective.*

Hepatitis B vaccine works well in preventing HBV infection and should be given to all who are at risk, such as male homosexuals (those who had not yet developed antibodies against HBV on their own) and medical personnel. If it were possible to give this vaccine worldwide, the incidence of liver cancer and cirrhosis of the liver would both be drastically reduced.

---

*Because regular immune globulin has too little anti-hepatitis B virus activity, donors who have been immunized against hepatitis B are the source of the gamma globulin used for individuals exposed to hepatitis B a few days before. This material is called hepatitis B immune globulin.

Hepatitis C

About 90 percent of cases of hepatitis diagnosed after blood transfusions and 12 to 15 percent of viral hepatitis not caused by HAV or HBV are caused by hepatitis C virus (HCV). Only about 4 percent of hepatitis C cases result from blood transfusions. The source of HCV infection in many patients is unknown. An authority on viral hepatitis* writes of exposure to contaminated needles in tattooing and acupuncture, and of needles and syringes in intravenous drug use. Perhaps even a single exposure, long forgotten, could lead to this infection, which would explain many of the unknowns.

The same author believes that the risk of maternal-fetal transmission is small and that sexual transmission is rare, so rare in fact that the Center for Disease Control advises that monogamous couples, in which one partner is infected with HCV, have no need to use condoms or to modify their sexual practices.

Many cases of HCV infection start clinically with the same pattern described for almost all the virus/hepatitis patients previously, but for hepatitis C these signs and symptoms are usually mild. A good number of cases of HCV infection are so mild as to go unrecognized by the patient. In the general population 0.13 to 1.7 percent will test positive for HCV infection.

Clinically, hepatitis C is usually a mild illness, but

---

*T. F. Bader, M.D., *Viral Hepatitis* (Seattle: Hogrefe and Huber, 1997).

about half the HCV infections become chronic, lasting beyond six months. After several years some of these may clear spontaneously, and others may remain benign, but about 30 percent of the chronic cases go on to develop cirrhosis of the liver, a scarring of the liver where cells have been destroyed. Some may then develop liver cell cancer, but only after cirrhosis has first been present.

It may take as long as six months from the time of exposure for HCV to present itself, but most often the incubation period is from six to nine weeks. Identifying blood tests may not become positive until long after the illness has begun. Contagiousness starts one or more weeks before the illness does, persists through the acute illness and, in those remaining chronically infected, continues indefinitely.

Interferon, an antivirus substance our bodies produce, given to treat acute hepatitis C may reduce the risk of chronic hepatitis C developing, but its usefulness is not yet established. The value of immune globulin in aborting illness after exposure to HCV is also not certain. An antivirus preparation that is now being tried (Intron A®, known to science as interferon alpha-2b) may have some value in treating chronic carriers, but otherwise, treatment is given only to relieve symptoms. On 3 million units of Intron A® I.V. administered three times per week, 69 percent of eighty patients improved whereas only 11 percent of ninety-seven controls did.

Hepatitis D

Even among viruses—a strange lot to begin with—
hepatitis D virus (HDV), also known as the delta virus,
is most peculiar. It can only infect a person if the hepatitis B virus attacks with it, which is known as a coinfection or if HBV infection is already present, a superinfection with HDV can occur, i.e., an infection with HDV on
top of the preexisting HBV infection. By itself, however,
HDV is powerless.

A coinfection will ordinarily produce a mild illness,
as though HBV alone were present, but the destruction
of the liver that is unusual in the case of acute HBV
infection alone becomes more common when HDV is
also present. Superinfection with HDV may lead to a
severe flare-up of chronic hepatitis or bring on an acute
case in asymptomatic carriers of HBV.

In the United States most cases of HDV infection
occur through the use of contaminated needles or
syringes for drug injections or from receiving multiple
blood transfusions. Hemophiliacs receiving blood-derived products are also at risk. Because HBV must also
be present for infection with HDV to occur, the possibility of sexual transmission also exists. In the countries
surrounding the Mediterranean, HDV infection is very
common and appears to be spread by close personal
contact.

Hepatitis D is diagnosed by determining the existence of HDV antibodies.

Hepatitis E

Except for one very important aspect, hepatitis E virus (HEV) infection is very like HAV infection: The illness tends to be mild, the patient does not become a carrier, but, sadly, if a woman in the last three months of pregnancy catches it, she stands about a one in five chance of dying of the HEV infection. Fortunately, HEV is rarely encountered in the United States.

Fecally contaminated water is the usual source of infection, but the fecal-oral route probably operates for person-to-person transmission (for example, putting unwashed hands in the mouth or contaminating food with unwashed hands). The possibility of sexual transmission exists (via anal-oral contact), but confirmatory evidence has been lacking.

The period of communicability is not known but is probably similar to that of HAV.

Although gamma globulin is effective in the treatment of HAV, that is not the case here. Instead, treatment consists of medication directed against bothersome symptoms.

11

Sexually Transmitted Diseases You Just Can't Stomach

Many diseases of the gastrointestinal tract frequently associated with spoiled or poorly prepared food or contaminated water can also be transmitted through sexual contact. Anilingus, stimulating the anal region with the lips and tongue for erotic pleasure (what is colloquially known as "rimming"), is the vehicle for this type of transmission. The organisms that cause these intestinal diseases are present in the stool, and traces of stool, visible or invisible, are present in the anal region.

A rundown on the most common of these exotically acquired conditions would include amebiasis, giardiasis, salmonellosis, shigellosis (also known as bacillary dysentery), campylobacter enteritis, and enterobiasis.

These names are unfamiliar in most homes but are associated with distressingly familiar signs and symptoms, diarrhea and abdominal distress, which come with most of them.

These illnesses are found mostly in male homosexuals when sexually acquired, but they can also afflict heterosexuals who venture into oral-anal pleasures without a barrier, such as plastic wrap, a dental dam, or a condom cut open down its length, between the mouth and anus.

Let's check out the early characteristic features of these sexually transmitted intestinal conditions, one at a time. (For each of these diseases, sexual partners of those infected should be tested for infection, especially if there has been any anal-oral contact.)

Amebiasis*

Amebiasis is caused by *Entamoeba histolytica*, a one-celled creature known as a protozoan. It is ordinarily spread by taking in fecally contaminated food or water, but in some instances infection of the vulva, cervix, and penis point to sexual transmission. In the past twenty years or so, studies have implicated anilingus as a major mode of transmission, as the male homosexual community exhibits a high level of carriers.

The incubation period extends from a few days to a few months.

---

*(a''-mee-beye'-à-sis)

Many carriers do not exhibit any symptoms, and others may have the mildest of abdominal discomforts, but some may have infections so severe as to cause frequent bloody diarrhea. More typical is a recurrent diarrhea accompanied by cramps but without visible blood.

Diagnosis is made by microscopic examination of stool specimens for active forms of the *Entamoeba histolytica* or inactive cysts.

Patients who may have an amoebic infection are treated with chemotherapeutic agents (chemicals used in treating infections, cancer, and other conditions) and, occasionally, with an added antibiotic (therapeutic agents derived from fungi, bacteria, or other organisms). Follow-up stool examinations are needed for proof of cure.

Sexual partners should also be checked.

Giardiasis*

Giardia lamblia, also a protozoan, is mainly a water-borne infectious agent, although a few cases of giardiasis are due to contaminated food. The organism usually infects the small intestine and may cause nausea, bloating, abdominal cramps, fatigue, weight loss, and chronic diarrhea. Most carriers have no symptoms.

The incubation period is about one to three weeks, although it may be longer. The disease remains infectious for a highly variable time.

---

*(jee"-ahr-dyé-à-sis)

Diagnosis is made by multiple microscopic studies of stool specimens, searching for the responsible organism. Sometimes a biopsy of the small intestine is needed to confirm the diagnosis.

Treatment is with chemotherapeutic agents. Follow-up stool examinations are important to ensure that cure has been achieved.

Salmonellosis*

Salmonella bacteria, of which there are about two thousand types, usually bring on a sudden illness characterized by headache, fever, nausea, occasional vomiting, abdominal pain, and bloody diarrhea, which lasts three to five days. Some strains of salmonella will bring on typhoid fever, or paratyphoid fever; others will invade the blood stream and settle in almost any section of the body. Many cases of salmonella, however, are so mild that there is no illness.

Pets as well as human beings may be the source of infection. Cleaning up the fecal matter of an infected pet can lead to infection if the hands are not washed. Eating inadequately cooked meat from infected food animals (such as chicken) or ingesting contaminated food or liquid are the two chief avenues of transmission. A small number of the estimated five million cases that occur in the United States each year are transmitted by oral-anal contact. Group outbreaks of the illness are usually

*(sal"-mà-nell-o'-sis)

caused by contaminated food; in individuals the source of the infection is not always clear.

The incubation period, usually twelve to thirty-six hours, may span six to seventy-two hours. The diagnosis is made by stool culture.

Ordinarily, the only treatment needed is the relief of symptoms, but if blood infection is suspected, antibiotics and chemotherapy may be used.

Bacillary Dysentery*

Bacillary dysentery, also known as shigellosis, is transmitted by contact, either direct or indirect, with infected stool. In homosexual males this frequently occurs as a result of oral-anal contact.

The shigella bacterium causes an illness with a rapid and unexpected onset, with fever, chills, loss of appetite, headache, and diarrhea with marked abdominal cramping, blood and mucus in one's stool, in addition to pus cells in microscopic quantities. Clinically, there is often marked dehydration and low blood pressure.

The incubation period may be as short as half a day or as long as seven days.

The diagnosis is made by culturing stool or swabs that have absorbed rectal fluids.

The symptoms are treated as needed, with intravenous fluids for low blood pressure, dehydration, electrolyte

*(bas'-i-la"-ree dis-àn-ter"-ee)

imbalances, and acidosis; antispasmodics for severe cramps; and medication to cut the frequency of bowel movements. Antibiotics and chemotherapeutic agents are used to eliminate the bacteria that cause this disease.

Campylobacter Enteritis*

The common clinical picture of an acute campylobacter bacterial infection includes diarrhea associated with fever, malaise, nausea, vomiting, and abdominal pain. Some infected people do not get sick at all. The illness usually lasts two to ten days, although it may hang on longer, and there may be relapses. Blood and pus cells may be found in the stool.

Diagnosis is made via stool culture.

Animals are the usual carriers. Contact with animal feces and subsequent failure to wash the hands thoroughly with soap and water (allowing the lather to remain on the skin at least fifteen seconds) and then handling or preparing food with soiled hands can lead to the spread of a campylobacter infection through ingestion of infected food. Raw milk and fecally contaminated water also are sources of infection. And, of course, oral-anal sex may lead to the infection as well.

The incubation period is one to ten days, and the illness remains communicable for up to three weeks.

Only in treating severe episodes are antibiotics used.

---

*(kam"-pà-low-bak'-tàr en-tà-reye'-tis)

*   *   *

Having dealt with oral-anal activity leading to intestinal diseases contracted during sexual activity, we now come to a condition once considered trivial, which at present weighs in as a threat to life: warts! If you're tempted to say, "You must be kidding," read through the next chapter to see what I mean.

12

The Bumpy Road

It used to be thought that all warts were caused by the same virus and that warts were no big deal, just nuisances. However, in 1954 it was established that genital warts were contagious. In 1977 an association was noted between flat warts (warts that are flush with the skin surface) and the appearance of precancerous changes in the cervix. That set off medical alarms that are still sounding, because some of those precancers became cancers, and the previous nuisance condition now called for early elimination. Affected women now require long-term surveillance, including annual physical examinations and Pap smears, which allow the physician to look for wart recurrences and newly developed precancerous and cancerous lesions.*

About sixty types of human papilloma virus (HPV) have been identified to date, and each has been assigned an identity number. Each of the types is specialized according to the sites it attacks and the kind of wart it produces. Type 1, for instance, is responsible for warts on the soles of the feet, and type 4 causes warts on the soles of the feet as well as on the palms.

Although warts are ordinarily benign skin and mucous membrane growths, genital warts are most often seen as cauliflower-like clusters of bunched slender stalks, caused by HPV types 6 and 11. These warts may also affect the respiratory tract and the vocal cords. Types 16 and 18 and several other types are found especially on the cervix, where there are flattened warts that may escape detection unless special techniques are used.† These same types are found in precancers and cancers not yet clinically visible.

A third kind of genital wart, a pimplelike form, tends

---

*A Papanicolaou smear (pap smear for short) is a smear made with material scraped gently from the surface of the uterine cervix and smeared on a slide, which is then immersed in a preservative solution. It is later stained with dyes and examined microscopically.

†To identify these types of HPV, the cervix is painted with a solution of 4 or 5 percent acetic acid (the same strength the grocer sells as white vinegar) which turns HPV-invaded cells white; then using a magnifying glass (a colposcope) the involved areas can be more exactly defined.

to appear on the shaft of the penis, the outer labia, or the region in front of the anus, all relatively dry areas.

In men, as in women, the most common genital wart is the cauliflower type. It appears initially on or about the head of the penis, where tiny traumatic abrasions from the friction of sexual intercourse may allow infections to take hold, and inside and outside the foreskin. During the course of infection the shaft of the penis, the scrotum, and the opening of the urethra may all become involved.

In women, the cauliflowerlike warts frequently appear first between the posterior ends of the labia majora (the outer lips of the vagina), eventually spreading over the entire vulva. In about 20 percent of cases the spread includes the area between the vulva and the anus. Any or all of the vagina may become involved.

Genital warts, the most common of the viral sexually transmitted diseases, occur about three times more often than active genital herpes type 2, and, of all the sexually transmitted diseases, only gonorrhea and chlamydia are more common.* Genital warts are almost always sexually transmitted. It is not certain whether contaminated towels or other articles may occasionally be responsible for a new infection.

The incubation period ranges from one to twenty months, and the condition remains communicable as long as lesions can be found, including those not visible

---

*Herpes, gonorrhea, and chlamydia will each be discussed in later chapters.

to the naked eye. The diagnosis is made by examining the warts either directly or at samples of their tissue under a microscope.

Warts may clear spontaneously, without leaving a trace, but when treatment is called for it involves direct destruction of all HPV-occupied cells. No oral or injectable medication that can do the job has been discovered, so caustic chemicals, laser beams, and freezing (by means of liquid nitrogen) are among the methods used. None is completely satisfactory, most are painful, and the need for repeated treatment is common, as is the scarring that occurs as a result of treatment.

Because warts are usually transmitted by direct contact, patients may transfer warts to new, previously uninfected areas on themselves. Spread of the virus may be reduced through the use of condoms or other barrier methods, and such methods should be used for at least six months after treatment seems to have destroyed all observable lesions.

Sexual partners of patients require examination, and, if necessary, treatment.

Molluscum Contagiosum*

The friendliest of all sexually transmitted diseases has to be molluscum contagiosum, a viral infection of the outer layer of the skin. With it comes no fever, no malaise, no

_____

*(moll-us'-kum kàn-tay'-jee-o'-sum)

long-term bad effects. Scratching at the mild itch, which is the only real discomfort caused by molluscum, may spread the lesions into new territory.

Molluscum contagiosum may be transferred to others directly by close contact with the lesions or, indirectly, through shared towels or other contaminated objects.

Typically, the lesions, which appear in small numbers, are little, dome-shaped, waxy, skin-colored bumps with a central depression resembling a tiny navel. An individual bump lasts only two or three months, and after two or three years the bumps stop appearing.

We have no magic bullet, no quick harmless medical cure, for molluscum, but the skin can be cleared by freezing the lesions, by scraping them off, or by treating them locally through the application of a caustic substance such as phenol, silver nitrate, iodine, and trichloroacetic acid. These methods may leave scars, whereas spontaneous clearing leaves unblemished skin.

In young adults (those roughly between the years of 18 and 28), this is a sexually transmitted disease, with most lesions concentrated about the genitals, the inner thighs, and the lower abdomen. In children and the elderly, the lesions are more likely to be on the face, neck, trunk, and upper extremities. In those with AIDS or other conditions associated with impaired immune systems, large numbers of molluscum lesions may appear on the head and neck.

The incubation period runs between one week and six months.

Chancroid*

Chancroid, caused by the bacterium *Haemophilus ducreyi*, is an acute, contagious, painful disease producing large sores in the anogenital region. It is not a common disease (several thousand cases per year in the United States) and prostitutes are frequently the source of the infection. The disease is more often seen in men than in women. The silver lining in this very dark cloud is the tendency of chancroid to restrict its damage to that region only. Most often transmitted sexually, it sometimes strays nonsexually, as onto a member of the medical team caring for a chancroid patient.

The incubation period is about three to seven days.

Chancroid starts with small painful pimples, which quickly break down into shallow soft ulcers with reddish, irregular, undermined borders. There may be marked subsurface destruction in the underlying tissues. Ulcers may coalesce. The lymph nodes in the groin enlarge and break down, releasing pus that may drain through the shiny, red, tense, overlying skin. Fresh areas of skin that contact the ulcers may also ulcerate.

In males, chancroid may cause enough scarring of the foreskin to make retracting it difficult or impossible. The disease process may perforate the urethra, causing urine to emerge from a new, misplaced orifice.

In women, the ulcers may be located inside the vagina and may not cause early symptoms, but they

---

*(chan-kroid')

may lead to painful urination, painful intercourse, and a vaginal discharge. Any external ulcers behave as they do in men.

In both men and women, if chancroid is contracted during anal intercourse, bleeding and pain may accompany bowel movements.

The diagnosis is largely based on the appearance of the ulcers, because securing a culture of *Haemophilus ducreyi* is difficult. Stained smears from the ulcers for microscopic study are not very helpful either, because there are so many other microorganisms in the sores.

The sooner a physician is consulted the less damage chancroid will be allowed to inflict. Furthermore, other sexually transmitted diseases frequently coexist with chancroid (herpes simplex, gonorrhea, syphilis, and HIV), and consulting a doctor early will allow these conditions to be diagnosed and treated as well.

Antibiotics or chemotherapeutic agents usually bring a cure. Be certain to follow the physician's instructions regarding treatment, check-ups (including laboratory tests), and when sexual activity may be resumed. All sexual contacts of a patient should be checked and treated if necessary. Any areas of skin (whether the patient's own or someone else's) that contact the ulcers should be washed with soap and water or one of the other cleansing materials mentioned earlier.

Granuloma Inguinale*

Involving only those body parts most often hidden from public view, granuloma inguinale (also known as Donovanosis) is a chronic, ulcer-producing, sexually transmitted, inflammatory condition of low communicability. It involves primarily the skin, mucous membranes, and lymph channels of the genitals and the perianal region, and occasionally the face and the mouth. It is probably spread by contact with existing ulcers. Granuloma inguinale is caused by *Calymattobacterium granulomatis,* a mouth-filling name for a tiny bacterium, and it differs from chancroid in that the ulcers are painless and stained smears of those ulcers frequently disclose the characteristic groups of microorganisms known as Donovan bodies, which cause granuloma inguinale. Donovan bodies are bacilli that invade certain white blood cells and reproduce there, forming clumps in the cell body.

After a widely varying incubation period of about eight to eighty days, a red pimple appears. It quickly breaks down to produce a bumpy-surfaced, relatively painless sore which spreads to adjacent areas. An assortment of other germs may secondarily invade the open areas, giving rise to a foul discharge from the denuded flesh and, with it, pain. The lymph nodes of groin areas are not usually involved, but the disease may generate lumps under the skin resembling nodes.

Ordinarily a disease of the tropics and subtropics, a

---

*(gran"-yà-low'-mà in"-gwàn-ahl)

small number of cases occur in the United States each year.

Early on the ulcers may look much like the lesions of syphilis, chancroid, and lymphogranuloma venereum (to be discussed later), and may even be mistaken for skin cancer. It is common for other sexually transmitted diseases (such as gonorrhea, syphilis, herpes, and HIV) to be present along with granuloma inguinale.

Examination and testing by a physician are required in order to sort out these possibilities. A tiny section of the involved tissue is removed, placed on a slide, and appropriately stained. Microscopic examination will disclose certain cells to be harboring groups of *Calymattobacterium microorganisms* (Donovan bodies), establishing the diagnosis.

Antibiotics or chemotherapeutic agents are used in treatment, which occasionally may take as long as three months to reach a cure.

Sexual partners should be examined and tested by a physician, but partners may lessen their chances of infection by washing with soap and water any areas that may have come in contact with an ulcer.

Again, the physician's advice should be adhered to as closely as possible. Follow-ups may last six months, but sexual activity may be resumed as soon as all ulcers are healed.

The scarring in the wake of granuloma inguinale occurs where the ulcers have been and may result in considerable long-lasting discomfort and disability, which vary greatly depending on how long the individual took to see a physician: Severe scarring can even lead to the inability to retract the foreskin and pass urine. The earlier the treatment is begun, the better the result.

13

A Clammy Feeling

Chlamydia*

Chlamydia are unique microorganisms, not bacteria, that can only live within cells. They survive and reproduce by borrowing the cells' energy-processing machinery. In developing societies, almost all chlamydia infections are sexually transmitted except in infants.

It is only in very recent years that we have been able to isolate and identify chlamydia as the cause of about half the cases of nongonorrheal urethritis (previously

---

*(klà-mid'-ee-à)

also known as nonspecific urethritis or nonspecific genital infections) in men.

Nongonorrheal urethritis is typically described as an awareness of the urethra not normally present, sometimes a soreness, with frequent painful voiding and a clear or opaque, pus-filled discharge. Some men, on waking in the morning, find the opening of the urethra glued shut by dried discharge. Later complications may include scarring of the urethra, causing narrowing of the urinary stream and inflammation of deeper genital structures, such as the urethra, cervix, salpinx, and epididymis.

Most women develop no symptoms from an early infection with *Chlamydia trachomatis*, but those who do may have frequent painful urination, vaginal discharge, pelvic pain, and pain during intercourse. Inflammation of mouth and rectum may follow intercourse at those sites, with sore throat and painful defecation.

Chlamydia infection may result in severe complications in many women. Inflammation of the lining of the uterus and fallopian tubes and pelvic inflammatory disease (PID) caused by chlamydia, will lead to infertility in about half the women who have had at least three episodes. (About one in five patients, both male and female, will relapse and require retreatment one or more times.) The most frequent cause of female infertility in this country is probably chlamydial infection, which displaced gonorrhea in that ranking in the United States. Acute inflammation and cyst formation of Bartholin's glands (the lubricating glands close to the entrance to the vagina) are other chlamydial complications.

The disease usually develops about one to four weeks after exposure through sexual intercourse with an infected individual. A variety of laboratory tests, some on the leading edge of technology, may be needed to clinch the diagnosis. If the laboratory facilities are not adequate (as is the case in some communities), patients are frequently treated on the basis of a presumptive diagnosis.

The treatment of chlamydial infections requires appropriate antibiotic or chemotherapeutic agents. Sexual partners must also be examined and treated.

Lymphogranuloma Venereum*

It's very likely that you have never, or rarely, heard of lymphogranuloma venereum. A highly contagious sexually transmitted disease with ugly consequences, lymphogranuloma venereum is caused by a few subtypes of *Chlamydia trachomatis*, different from those that cause many of the cases of nongonococcal urethritis (inflammation of the urethra not caused by the gonorrheal germ) and pelvic inflammatory disease. The disease is seldom encountered in the United States, but it does occur in parts of Asia, Africa, South America, the Caribbean, and other warm regions. If you are planning a trip to any of these places, and your plans include sexual adventuring, lymphogranuloma venereum should be of special interest to you.

---

*(lim"-fà-gran-yà-ló-mà và-neer'-ee-àm)

A few cases of lymphogranuloma venereum are spread nonsexually, as by direct and indirect contact with fluid from the sores that it causes, but most of the small number of cases appearing in the United States result from sexual contact with a person from the tropics or subtropics.

Between roughly three and thirty days after exposure, a small painless blister, pimple, or ulcer will appear briefly on the penis or labia, behind the vulva, or within the vagina. This lesion clears without leaving a scar, and may cause so little trouble it may not be noticed. Anywhere from a few weeks to as long as six months later, the lymph nodes connected with the area first involved will enlarge and fill with pus. In heterosexual males, the enlarged nodes are usually where they can be seen and felt, in the groin area. But in females, homosexual males, and, occasionally, heterosexual males, they are sometimes found around the rectum, where they are usually invisible.

The glands break down and the pus drains through nearby surfaces through multiple disease-induced openings, scarring the region. In males the pus usually drains through the skin where the front of the thigh joins the trunk. In females the pus may flow into the rectum, vagina, bladder, large or small intestine, or the skin around the anus. In fact, more than one of these areas may be involved simultaneously. Blood may be mixed with the pus leaking through these openings. In males whose rectums are involved, the routes of discharge may be the same as in the female except, of course, that there is no vaginal exit.

Although mainly a disease of lymph channels and lymph nodes, the inflammation may also involve the adjacent tissues. Chills, fever, loss of appetite, joint pain, and headaches are common. Occasionally the destructive process involves other regions of the body.

The physician, after taking a history and performing an examination, will depend on the pattern of symptoms and objective findings and a few refined blood tests to establish the diagnosis. Tests for syphilis and other sexually transmitted diseases will probably be done, with the physician's follow-up lasting up to six months.

To kill the causative bacteria, antibiotics or chemotherapeutic agents are used. Often, within two to four weeks, the physician will find clearing of the lesions and will give the go-ahead for resumption of sexual activity.

Unfortunately, the scarring left by the active disease cannot be undone, and it may lead to enough blockage of lymph drainage to cause chronic swelling of the genitals and, rarely, the legs. Some of the complications from scarring may require surgery for their correction.

It should be immediately apparent that earlier diagnosis and treatment lead to better long-term results. It is equally apparent that avoiding situations of contact with the disease is even better.

14

Syphilis

Syphilis,* which is caused by a spiral slender bacterium known as a spirochete (specifically, *Treponema pallidum*), can destroy any and all organs and tissues in our body. During the incubation period of anywhere from one to thirteen weeks, the spirochetes spread throughout the body. Untreated syphilis proceeds through several stages, but we will deal mostly with the readily contagious primary and secondary stages. Syphilis is rarely contagious once it has progressed beyond the second stage.

A chancre, the primary lesion, starts as a small, red

---

*(sif'-à-lis)

pimple on the spot where the spirochete entered the body. It soon becomes an enlarging, painless nontender, highly contagious sore, with a firm raised border. The chancre may appear on the penis, on or in the female genitalia, on the anus, or in the rectum, or anywhere on the body. If untreated the sore lasts four to eight weeks before clearing completely on its own. Some individuals have more than one chancre, and in some persons infection may be established without any chancre being observed.

In about a quarter of the cases, the second stage begins while the chancre is still present. This stage involves widespread enlargement of lymph nodes, which are nontender and firm; headache; loss of appetite; nausea; generalized aching; easy tiring; low-grade fever; neck stiffness; and other symptoms indicative of total body involvement. An assortment of symmetrically distributed rashes, which may resemble the rashes seen in other diseases, appears on the skin and mucous membranes. A somewhat unusual feature is the presence of a rash on the palms and soles, which most rashes spare. Ordinarily there is no itching. The rashes may appear in crops that clear up and recur for up to a few years. They may be flush with the skin, be tiny bumps, be scaly, or appear as pus pimples.

In the mouth and on other mucous membranes, such as in the vagina and rectum, mucous patches appear as grayish, circular, red-bordered areas swarming with microscopic spirochetes.

In moist, warm areas, where skin rests or rubs (such as around the anus, vulva, scrotum, armpits, inner thighs, under heavy breasts or stout abdomen, or in the webs between fingers and toes) grayish, moist, flat areas that are slightly elevated above the skin's surface develop. These areas are called *condylomata lata* and they are loaded with spirochetes.

Syphilis is transmitted when an intact mucous membrane or abraded skin comes in contact with mucous patches; *condylomata lata*; the semen, blood, or vaginal discharges of a patient with secondary syphilis; or the wet chancre of primary syphilis.

Other illnesses may present signs and symptoms that resemble syphilis, but the physician will be able to distinguish it from other illnesses by taking a history of the patient and performing a blood test. Treatment with an antibiotic will cure syphilis, but the physician may want to follow the patient for months afterward for observation and further testing.

During the primary stages of syphilis all persons sexually contacted during the three months prior to diagnosis should be examined and treated if necessary. If the disease is not diagnosed until it has reached the secondary stage, this period should be extended to six months.

Unfortunately, some people have such mild primary and secondary syphilis that the signs and symptoms are ignored. Spontaneous clearing of these two stages occurs and the syphilis goes "underground." It may then, years later, lead to severe organ system damage, disability, and premature death.

15

Gonorrhea

Gonorrhea* (clap, as it is known in some circles) is an acute sexually transmitted infection caused by a bacterium, *Neisseria gonorrhea*. It may produce an inflammation of the inner lining of the urethra, cervix, and other, deeper, structures of the female and male reproductive tracts. The rectum, the eyes, and the pharynx may also be involved. Infrequently the bacteria may get into the blood stream and spread to other sites in the body, including the joints, the inner lining of the heart, the surface of the liver, and the membranes surrounding the brain.

---

*(gon"-à-reé-à)

In addition to the disagreeable consequences that may result from gonorrhea invading the blood, sterility, ectopic pregnancy, internal abscess requiring surgery, and scarring of the urethra leading to difficulty voiding are some of the other serious complications that may result from gonorrhea.

After contracting gonorrhea, about 80 percent of females and about 60 percent of males have few or no symptoms, allowing the infection to go unnoticed until characteristic symptoms develop in a sexual partner. At that point the asymptomatic individual who is the source of the infection can be traced and identified.

About three million cases of gonorrhea occur in the United States each year, 90 percent of them in teenagers and young adults. About 250 million cases occur each year worldwide.

After an incubation period of two to fourteen days, those males who develop symptoms will experience a mild itching or burning discomfort, progressing to painful urination and a frequent urgent need to void immediately. This should be an indication that something abnormal is going on. A yellowish-green discharge from the urethra soon appears, as does a reddening of the urethral opening.

In the female it may take one to three weeks for symptoms, which are mostly mild, to develop (itching and burning), but sometimes painful and frequent urination and an increased vaginal discharge occur. These initial manifestations, in both sexes, should be taken as a clear call for medical consultation.

Unrecognized gonorrhea is not transmitted in

straightforward vaginal intercourse if a properly used condom is employed during vaginal and rectal intercourse and fellatio. Fellatio without condom use that is performed on an infected male will frequently result in gonorrhea of the throat. On the other hand, cunnilingus on an infected female only occasionally results in gonorrhea of the throat, and even that small incidence may be prevented by interposing a rubber dental dam or household plastic wrap between mouth and vulva.

According to various estimates in the medical literature, a single exposure of unprotected sexual intercourse with an infected male results in the female's contracting gonorrhea 50 to 80 percent of the time. The infected male's ejaculate, containing numerous gonorrhea germs, may linger in the vagina for hours after intercourse, thus increasing the female's exposure to the germs. This represents another instance of life's unfairness to women, because males who have unprotected intercourse with an infected female get gonorrhea only 20 to 30 percent of the time.*

Gonorrhea may also be transmitted through non-sexual means: Young girls may pick up pelvic gonorrhea from contaminated towels, panties, or even a toilet seat moist with gonorrheal pus. Even so, sexual molestation must also be considered a possibility in infants and young girls who develop gonorrhea.

---

*See J. M. Reinisch, *The Kinsey Institute New Report on Sex* (New York: St. Martin's, 1990), and J. D. McKloskey, *Your Sexual Health* (San Francisco: Halo Books, 1993).

Another nonsexual form of transmission, a contaminated finger touching an eye, could cause an acute gonorrheal eye inflammation that may result in serious eye damage if it is not treated quickly.

The possibility of such transmission explains why all newborns are given prophylactic eyedrops right after birth: Some mothers may have an unrecognized gonorrheal or other infection of the birth canal that may get into the baby's eyes during delivery.

In more than 90 percent of males, gonorrhea is diagnosed after microscopic examination of the stained smear of material from the urethra. In females, however, smears yield an accurate diagnosis only about 60 percent of the time. Therefore, in females, and the 10 percent of males with nondiagnostic smears, cultures have to be done to ensure accuracy of diagnosis.

About one-quarter of heterosexual males with gonorrheal urethritis (inflammation of the urethra caused by gonorrhea) will also be infected with *Chlamydia trachomatis*, and 25 to 50 percent of women with gonorrheal urethritis will also have a *Chlamydia trachomatis* infection. Only 5 to 10 percent of homosexual men with gonorrhea will have a coinfection with chlamydia. Chlamydia, however, may produce an illness clinically resembling gonorrhea but slower in onset and in full development.

Treatment of gonorrhea has become more complicated in recent years because strains of the gonococcus that are resistant to penicillin, previously an almost sure-cure agent, have evolved. Alternative antibiotic and chemotherapeutic treatments are available to patients.

Because gonorrhea and chlamydia so often travel together (they apparently favor the same environment), many doctors will treat for both when they find or suspect one of the two diseases. Unfortunately the agents for treating gonorrhea will not cure a chlamydia infection, which requires a different set of medications. Doctors reason that the risks involved in treating unnecessarily are minor compared with the damage that could result from nontreatment during days that will pass while waiting for culture reports.

After proving cure by posttreatment examination and testing, the physician will approve resumption of sexual intercourse.

Recurrences usually indicate a fresh infection rather than a relapse.

16

Herpes Simplex and Related Diseases

Herpes Simplex

Before there was AIDS there was herpes, remember? Herpes simplex of itself is rarely life-endangering in otherwise healthy adults, but herpes simplex virus type-2 was, and remains, one of the most dreaded of sexually transmitted diseases. Why? Because its recurrent attacks impose days-to-weeks-long periods of unhappy abstinence on sexually active individuals. A real downer!

But that is getting ahead of our story.

Herpes simplex is a virus with a moderately severe primary infection and clinically milder recurrences. In other words, the initial occurrence of the disease is usually the worst. Subsequent flare-ups are not as severe as the first attack.

There are two types of herpes simplex virus (HSV) that cause herpes simplex infections: HSV-type 1 (HSV-1) and HSV-type 2 (HSV-2). The two differ a little in their chemical makeup and behavior, but the skin lesions they produce are identical.

HSV-1 does its mischief mostly in and around the mouth, and, to a lesser degree, anywhere above the waist. HSV-2 usually operates below the waist, mainly in the genito-anal region and the nearby skin.

In the past twenty or thirty years, as more and more of us have discovered the joys of oral-genital sex, and some even oral-anal sex, more HSV-1 infections have appeared below the waist and HSV-2 above the waist.

Their behavior is altered in their transplanted sites. HSV-1 infection, which may recur about the mouth frequently for years, particularly after exposure to stresses, such as fever, trauma, or certain foods and medicines, may infect the genital region and recur only once or not at all. A primary infection with HSV-2 below the waist will recur in 60 to 80 percent of those individuals. However, HSV-2 infection about the mouth will recur less frequently there than HSV-1 does. In general, with the passage of time, HSV infections tend to recur less frequently.

A typical episode usually begins with itching, tingling, aching, or other discomfort over a small area of skin or mucous membrane, lasting a few hours or up to a few days. Then a crop of tiny blisters appears in the same area, on a reddened base. The blisters break, leaving open sores oozing a liquid teeming with the virus. A fingertip moistened by that fluid may cause a loss of vision in an eye infected by the finger. If the finger has even a tiny abrasion where the fluid from the blister has touched, the finger itself may develop a herpes infection. Moisture from the raw surface of broken herpes blisters can establish new sites of herpes infection anywhere on the body if a small break in the skin gives the virus particles in the fluid a portal of entry.

A yellowish crust soon forms over the blister liquid. When the crust has all fallen off, days later, the episode is considered over.

The primary infection, in addition to the sequence described above, may be accompanied by fever, malaise, and enlarged lymph nodes. The entire first episode sometimes lasts up to three weeks and is more severe and somewhat longer than the recurrences.

A diagnosis for herpes is made by culturing fluid from the blisters or ulcers; blood tests are not sufficiently reliable.

HSV infections last a lifetime, and many individuals remain unaware of their infection. They may transmit the virus to a partner even while free of any manifestation of disease, but shedding of the virus (transmission through body fluids expelled from any of the body's orifices) and spread of the disease is much more likely at times of clinical activity and probably for several days afterward.

Although the incubation period is officially one to twenty days, the disease usually presents in six to eight days.

By the time they reach age ten, about 90 percent of the population of the United States has been infected with HSV-1, through kissing or by droplets from a sneeze or cough. Of these, 20 to 40 percent suffer recurrences.*

Herpes simplex virus type-2 causes 85 to 95 percent of genital herpes and is acquired by most people through sexual activity when they are between the ages of fifteen and forty-five. Inanimate objects, such as wet towels and toilet seats, are rarely involved in transmission of herpes.

It is important to see a physician with the first appearance of herpes. Other diseases, including some that are sexually transmitted, may resemble herpes (e.g., syphilis, shingles), and it takes a physician's examination and testing to determine what is going on. The physician's experience will determine what is the best available treatment.

At the present time there is no cure for herpes, but medications that may shorten an attack or cut down on the frequency of recurrences are available.

As with other sexually transmitted diseases, the partner of a patient should also consult a physician.

---

*See M. A. Krupp and M. Chatton, *Current Medical Diagnosis and Treatment* (Los Altos: Lange Medical Publications, 1982), p. 345, and A. Benenson, *Control of Communicable Disease in Man* (Washington, D.C.: American Public Health Association, 1990), p. 213.

Cytomegalovirus* Infection

Cytomegalovirus (CMV) is a virus in the herpes family which is spread by contact with infected body fluids. The virus has been found in saliva, urine, semen, cervical secretions, maternal milk, and in blood and blood-derived products. About 60 to 70 percent of adults have been infected by CMV, which probably remains in the body for a lifetime (it may be shed in saliva and urine for years).

A small number of fetuses and newborns may suffer severe or fatal damage from CMV picked up in the uterus, or by feeding on their mother's milk, but most babies remain asymptomatic, with a few having only a positive urine culture to show the CMV infection.

Some of the adult CMV infections are sexually acquired. Primary infection in adults, which has an incubation period of twenty to sixty days, may cause no symptoms, or may show up as fever, malaise, and generalized aching, sometimes with a rash or with a liver inflammation detectable with liver function tests. All symptoms clear up in two or three weeks.

In the case of CMV infection there are no enlarged lymph nodes or sore throat such as many patients get with infectious mononucleosis (which will be discussed shortly), which, clinically, closely resembles CMV infection. Both illnesses develop unusual-looking white blood cells, but only infectious mononucleosis tests positive in a certain blood test.

---

*(sigh"-toe-meg"-à-low-vye'-ràs)

In otherwise healthy adults, CMV illness is benign and self-limited, with only really bothersome symptoms calling for treatment.

A CMV infection in those with an impaired immune system, however, may develop with a ferocity that could cause bodily damage and death. Those most likely to be severely affected include organ-transplant recipients, whose immune systems have been deliberately suppressed to prevent rejection of the new organ, or those suffering from an infection (such as HIV) that has damaged the immune system. The CMV then reinforces the HIV, further damaging the immune system.

One of the most dreaded consequences of an out-of-control CMV infection is an inflammation of the retina, resulting in blindness. Although we have no cure for a CMV infection, we do have a few antiviral agents that may avert blindness or even CMV's threat to life. These therapeutic agents must be continued for the patient's lifetime.

When CMV virus is found in urine, it may have been present in urine, by way of chronic shedding, for years. We now have tests that tell us whether the virus in the urine is really a persistent trace from an old CMV infection or whether it is a brand new CMV infection. If it is not a new CMV infection, then the illness is probably due to some other disease.

Any illness that suggests by its signs and symptoms that it might be a sexually transmitted disease calls for quick consultation with a physician.

Infectious Mononucleosis

Is open mouth-to-mouth kissing (also known as French kissing) a form of sexual intercourse? If yes, then infection with the Epstein-Barr virus (EBV), also known as infectious mononucleosis, mono, glandular fever, or the kissing disease, is definitely a sexually transmitted disease, even though genital transmission appears to be rare.

Nonsexual transmission is common among children, probably by way of saliva-contaminated food or other materials a young child, or infant, puts in its mouth. Half the individuals in the United States have picked up the Epstein-Barr virus by age five; the early infection rate is even higher in less-developed countries.

Epstein-Barr virus, one of the herpes-virus group, is very selective about the cells it attacks: B cells (the cells that produce protective antibodies), the lining cells of the nose and upper throat, and the lining cells of the uterine cervix.

In individuals infected under age ten, any illness that results from an EBV infection is mild. Of those who pick the virus up from age ten into early adulthood, about half will become ill with infectious mononucleosis. The incubation period is given as anywhere from five days to six weeks, depending on the text you consult.

The illness is often characterized by an inflammation of the tonsils and pharynx, swelling of the lymph nodes, particularly those at the back of the neck, and an assortment of laboratory abnormalities: a white-blood-cell count with at least 10 percent of abnormal cells; a positive

heterophile antibody test (a blood test especially designed to pick up infectious mononucleosis); and, in
about 95 percent of cases, liver-function-test abnormalities, although only one in about twenty-five patients will
become jaundiced. Along with these symptoms there
will be fever lasting from days up to several weeks,
malaise, muscle aches, and loss of appetite. Some
patients have minimal symptoms, and some will have a
long-lasting debility after the acute illness.

As with the other viruses, there is no medical cure.
The illness is self-limited and usually requires only the
relief of symptoms, although in some severely ill
patients, corticosteroids may be tried.

17

HIV and AIDS

Acquired immunodeficiency syndrome (AIDS) is a fatal condition caused by infection with the human immunodeficiency virus (HIV). HIV infection leads to damage of the immune mechanisms, the system designed by nature to protect us from bacteria, viruses, and other organisms and substances that are foreign and potentially harmful to our body.

In the United States the first cases of AIDS were recognized in 1981. Later the HIV virus was identified as the cause of the disease. HIV may have started in Africa where it is largely transferred heterosexually. In the United States the earliest AIDS patients were mostly male homosexuals or were intravenous drug users who shared syringes and needles among themselves without bothering to sterilize the equipment between uses.

In 1996 the number of New York City residents living with HIV/AIDS was about 128,700. Using the New York City statistics and knowing that health authorities calculate that New York City has one-sixth of all the HIV/AIDS cases in the United States, one can approximate the following national figures*:

Living with HIV/AIDS	772,200
Men	567,600
Women	180,000
Children	18,000
Deaths	26,400

Some people see AIDS as God's punishment for humankind's wicked ways. Scientists view it as another newly erupted epidemic on the world scene, similar to previous, frightening, rapidly spreading contagions such as the Black Death of the Middle Ages and the rampant influenza of 1918–1919, which resulted in about twenty million deaths.

The virus that causes AIDS can be transmitted, either directly or indirectly, even before symptoms of the disease have presented themselves. Directly, infection occurs when the virus-bearing body fluids of a carrier transfer to a partner through a break in the skin or

---

*Based on figures in *City Health Information* (New York City Department of Health), vol. 15, no. 4 (December 1996).

mucous membranes. (It isn't known if the virus is able to penetrate intact mucous membranes, as of the vagina, or rectum, or mouth, as it does the intact chimpanzee vagina.) What body fluids are we talking about? Blood, semen, and the lubricating fluid that leaks from the penis during sexual arousal (pre-cum) all contain the virus in amounts sufficient to cause infection. The female's blood, including menstrual blood, vaginal fluids, and breast milk are also hazardous. A woman who has HIV or acquires it during pregnancy can pass the virus on to her unborn child, and about 18 to 40 percent of such pregnancies do result in HIV-infected newborns. Those children who are lucky enough to escape HIV infection while in utero, however, may acquire it while nursing on their mother's HIV-infected breast milk. A woman may also transmit the virus to a sexual partner who sucks on her lactating breast.

But known HIV-positive pregnant women who receive antiviral therapy will have about a one-third reduction in children born infected with HIV. About 500 HIV-infected babies are born in the United States annually (as of 1997). About 1,000 a day are born in the developing countries.* Open-mouth kissing, with exchange of saliva, had not been confirmed as a source of infection, but in 1997 one such case in the United States was reported (after all, some gums do bleed easily). Any fluid, such as saliva or urine, not usually considered a danger, becomes a threat with blood in it.

---

*Associated Press, Sept. 4, 1997.

Indirect transmission occurs via injections, using blood-contaminated needles or syringes, or by sharing sex toys, enema or douching equipment, razors or toothbrushes, or any objects that might possibly be exposed to a carrier's blood. Blood transfusions and blood-derived products, such as plasma, platelets, and packed white blood cells as are used in treating hemophiliacs, caused many cases of HIV infection before testing developed enough to improve the safety of the blood supply.

Two to four weeks after being infected with HIV, fewer than half the people involved will suffer from a nondescript illness characterized by malaise, fever, and joint pains lasting three to fourteen days, and enlarged lymph nodes, which may persist long after the other discomforts have cleared. Many of these individuals then join the majority of those newly infected with HIV in enjoying a long "honeymoon" of freedom from symptoms, for as long as ten or more years.

One to three months after a person's system is invaded by HIV, blood testing may disclose antibodies the body creates to fight against the virus, but sometimes it takes six months or even up to a few years before the test becomes positive. In 1997 we are at the leading edge of the development of a testing method that will identify an HIV infection within days of its onset, but as of this writing the test is not generally available yet.

For a time there was panic over being near anyone with AIDS or HIV infection. We know now that casual contact does not cause any new HIV infections if there is no exchange of body fluids, the disease cannot be transmitted. School, the workplace, social gatherings or other such contacts, or even living twenty-four hours a day with infected people (say, family members, for example) are perfectly safe.

It's important to understand that shaking hands; the droplets from sneezes or coughs; eating from the same plate; using the same phone, bathtub, or toilet seat; hugging; massaging; and social kissing on the cheeks or with closed lips will *not* result in the spread of HIV infections. Mosquitoes and other insects do not transmit HIV. Unprotected sexual intercourse or other intimacies, including sucking on the lactating breast of an HIV carrier by her partner or her infant, are highly risky activities, however.

The insidious damage of HIV eventually surfaces in the AIDS-Related Complex (ARC) comprising some, or all, of a group of signs, symptoms, and laboratory abnormalities, which usually precede the characteristic infections and tumors that identify AIDS itself. ARC includes malaise, weight loss (which may be severe), fatigue, recurrent fever, diarrhea, low white cell and platelet counts, anemia, and thrush (a yeast infection of the mouth).

Some patients die of ARC, but most go on to develop AIDS, and many skip ARC and go directly to AIDS, which is marked by the appearance of opportunistic infections: infections involving organisms that were previously benign but have become aggressive, widespread, and even lethal in the face of the immune system's dwindling ability to fight them off. For example, *Pneumocystis carinii,* a protozoan that is a gentle, easily contained organism in someone with an intact immune system, becomes life-threatening, and frequently a killer, when HIV has damaged the immune system sufficiently to allow the organism to produce pneumonia. Even the cells of lazy, slow-growing, malignant tumors, such as Kaposi's sarcoma,* may opportunistically charge wildly about the body. Any organ system, any part of the body, including the brain, may be involved in AIDS.

We still have no wonder pill to cure virus infections, but some of the antiviral drugs we do have may slow the damage caused by HIV. It is definitely worthwhile for individuals infected with HIV to see a doctor familiar with the management of HIV infection at regular intervals, even while feeling wonderful. The doctor, through appropriate testing, can determine when antiviral medication is called for. During these regular checkups, the doctor might note early clinical manifestations of one of the diseases in the AIDS-related complex and be able to nip the condition in the bud. Much can be done for individual components of the AIDS complex, particularly in

---

*Kaposi's sarcoma is a rare malignant tumor, displayed as bluish-red nodules on the skin or mucous membranes. It had occurred mostly in elderly white males in the USA until the arrival of the AIDS epidemic. Before AIDS it was only slowly progressive. It has become a rapidly progressive tumor in AIDS patients, involving the lungs and gastrointestinal tract as well as the skin, and appearing in younger individuals.

their early stages, and an impending disaster may be warded off, thereby extending the person's life. The AIDS complex comprises many infections and tumors in an individual with HIV, which may be mild and quiescent until the level of certain immune cells drops too low; then CMV infection may flare up, herpes may rampage, the blood-vessel tumor that is called Kaposi's sarcoma can spread through the body, and *Pneumocystis carinii* produces a pneumonia that may kill the patient.

Laboratories around the world are working to find a vaccine that could prevent or perhaps modify the course of HIV infection, and they are looking for new strategies for slowing its progression to full-blown AIDS, as well as for better methods of attacking particular components of AIDS. Many antiviral drug treatments have been developed, but the cost is often prohibitive, keeping help out of the reach of millions of sufferers. Researchers are hard at work seeking new and less expensive ways to control HIV.

Prevention remains the best method of dealing with HIV and the drop in new HIV infections in male homosexual groups who have been taught less risky sexual behavior evidences this claim. The benefits of detailed safer sex and drug-use education for people at risk will be among the primary weapons for curbing the AIDS epidemic.

A Special Case: HIV Testing

At several points in this book I have mentioned HIV testing, along with testing for gonorrhea, syphilis, chlamydia, and so on. HIV testing, however, because of the repercussions of a positive test, is unique among common tests for disease.

Because the impact of a positive test may have such a shattering effect on so many aspects of a person's existence, counseling before the test, with explanation of the testing procedure and discussion of the implications of negative and positive results, is highly desirable. Discussion is even more important at the time when a positive test result is disclosed.

The test really involves two antibody tests, both of which are done on blood samples. The first test done does not recognize the presence of HIV in the body, but rather identifies the antibody defense the body has mounted against the virus. Unfortunately, false negative and false positive tests occasionally occur. To improve the reliability of a positive test, it is repeated. If it is again positive, a different sort of antibody test is done. If the test remains positive, it is reasonably certain that the person is carrying HIV.

If you know that you have been exposed to HIV, but the test is negative, it is possible that the virus was picked up too recently for the antibody tests to have become positive. In the event of a negative result, retesting should be done three months later, and, if still negative, repeated after another three months. Rarely, an individual will have HIV and be capable of transmitting it but will not develop antibodies for more than a year, but by six months the vast majority of infected people will have generated a positive test. Sometimes, after HIV infection has developed into full-blown AIDS, a previously positive test will become negative, but then the pattern of the illness would indicate what is going on. With the severity of the immunodeficiency at the AIDS stage, it may not be possible to elicit an immune response that was previously present; this response is needed to recognize an infection with HIV.

Some individuals may assume from repeated negative tests that they must be immune to contracting the HIV infection, but we don't know of any such fortunate resistance to the virus.

A confirmed positive test means your body has the virus responsible for AIDS in it, that you may infect others with it, and that there is a strong possibility you may develop AIDS-Related Complex (ARC) or Acquired Immunodeficiency Syndrome (AIDS) somewhere down the line. The disease, however, may take ten or more years to develop. In 1997 an aura of hope has replaced the gloom-and-doom certainty that a miserable, premature death comes with every positive test—the arrival on the HIV/AIDS battleground of a new category of therapeutic agents, called protease inhibitors, which suppress the multiplication of HIV particles, especially when added to two of the older agents, called nucleosides. This new approach has taken individuals who were dying and restored them to such health that they were able to return to work.

Unfortunately, of the approximately 150,000 people on this new regimen, 25 to 30 percent of AIDS patients either do not respond or respond for as long as a year or more and then the virus breaks through. Dr. Anthony Fauci, a leading HIV scientist, estimates the failure rate may reach 50 percent.

Given a positive test for HIV infection, a drastic lifestyle change may be needed. Alcohol intake, drug use, smoking, or any other practice that may further damage the immune system, as these do, will add to the damage done by the virus and hasten the development of AIDS. Exposure to further HIV by using contaminated needles and syringes or by having unprotected sex, even if both partners already have HIV, will also be harmful. So will stress, it is now known; therefore, it's advisable for individuals with impaired immune systems to master at least one of the many techniques for reducing stress.

Pregnant women are especially hard hit by a positive test. They may transmit the HIV to the fetus or, later on, to the baby via nursing. If they learn of a positive result in the first three months of pregnancy, they may consider having an abortion. An alternative now available to them is to take during pregnancy injections of antiviral drugs that may lessen the sizable percentage of newborns who contract HIV while in the uterus. Pregnancy tends to accelerate the appearance of AIDS in the mother, and newborns with HIV tend to reach the AIDS stage more quickly than most adults.

If it becomes known in your community that you are

HIV positive, you may encounter discrimination in obtaining housing, finding or keeping a job, in acceptance at medical facilities, in your school or social life, or in getting insurance. Although this discrimination is illegal, it may be widespread. Skillful counseling, if available, can appreciably reduce the impact of these various emotional crises. Counseling may have to extend over a period of time as new, and frequently overwhelming, problems—social, financial, physical, etc.—crop up.

Many people are still frightened of individuals who are HIV positive. These people haven't learned yet that casual contacts at work, in school, or at social events, are not avenues of transmission of HIV. The public's disregard of the fact that HIV transmission occurs only through intimate contact with body fluids and not through ordinary social closeness accounts for the severe prejudice to which known HIV-positive individuals are exposed almost everywhere they go.

This unjust ostracism by the public explains, at least in part, the reluctance of many individuals to be tested for HIV and is even more influential in creating the HIV-positive individual's determination to keep that status secret.

A few years ago, the surgeon general of the United States issued guidelines regarding the right of society to know about a person's HIV status. He held that, there being no vaccine to prevent it, and no way to cure it, it was federal policy that the confidentiality of the individual's health record be protected and access to it be strictly limited. There are some states that have estab-

lished their own policies that run counter to those of the
federal government. These states require the reporting
of positive tests to local health authorities so that they
may trace the individual's contacts and test and advise
their sexual partners. The problem with such a state
policy is that those who may have reason to believe that
they are infected will tend to avoid being tested. There
are now good reasons for reporting HIV-positive
patients to health departments. With our developing
ability to identify an HIV infection in its first several
days by detecting the virus itself or some component of
HIV, we can now attack HIV early and maximally. With
our new combined therapies, we can attempt to eradi-
cate the virus in an individual. It thus makes sense to
seek out all infected individuals and their partners for
testing and, if necessary, for treatment.

The reporting and case-finding of sexually transmitted diseases have a long history, but there has been
no scientific statistical study, using an untreated control
group and a treated trial group, to establish that seeking
out contacts and treating those who are positive are
valid ways to end an epidemic. The health departments
proceed as they do because it makes common sense.

Since 1985 when HIV testing became generally available, AIDS-advocacy groups have fought to protect
AIDS-infected and HIV-positive individuals from having
their status revealed because of the discrimination that
known positive testers face in the community. In 1997
many HIV-positive groups and AIDS patients have come
to realize the value of early treatment of HIV infections to

maintain well-being and to prolong the interval before AIDS shows up. Some of these groups and individuals have very recently done an about-face and now favor HIV testing for the benefit of individuals and communities. As of this writing twenty states have HIV reporting, and Florida and New Mexico may soon join them. Every state does require that AIDS be reported. The federal government is now advocating laws to make HIV testing and reporting mandatory for all jurisdictions.

The national government is currently using a stick-and-carrot approach to encourage cooperation in implementing federal legislation passed in 1996. The stick: federal AIDS funds will be withheld from states not counseling and testing pregnant women and not reducing the incidence of HIV in newborns. The carrot: the AIDS money will continue to flow.

Because of the trend to earlier treatment, every patient given a positive test result should consult as soon as possible with a physician experienced in HIV / AIDS and in sexually transmitted diseases. Since medicine and so many other important fields move so swiftly these days, it pays to keep an eye and an ear on the media daily.

In certain communities there are clinics at which testing is done anonymously, without any record of the name, social security number, or any other identifying information about the person being tested. The clinic issues a unique identification number which later enables that person, and no one else, to obtain the test result and counseling. The individual who tests positive

may then make a decision whether to inform sex partners, to adopt safer sex practices, or to inform emergency room doctors of his or her HIV status. Presumably
the counseling given at the time the positive result is disclosed will help the individual make socially responsible
decisions and enable him or her to deal better with the
many new problems in life that the diagnosis brings. It
should also inform the positive tester how to obtain further information and counseling in the community. Any
public health facility should be able to direct an inquirer
to available resources locally. At the time of this writing
there is a National AIDS Hotline, 1-800-342-AIDS, that
can direct you to local assistance.

Other clinics may test confidentially, in which case
the test result is strictly limited to certain medical personnel, but these are usually clerical workers, who may
talk about what they see. Such records may occasionally
be subpoenaed and become available to others.

In 1996 kits for testing yourself for HIV became com-
mercially available in most states. A private code enables
you to determine anonymously whether you have the
virus. Your follow-up on getting the result should be
expert counseling. As of 1997 there were two self-testing
kits on the market: Confide® provided by Direct Access
Diagnostics and Home Access® by Home Access Health
Care Corp. Confide® is available in major pharmacies as
a kit, costing $35.50 (in 1997). It provides equipment for
pricking a fingertip to obtain a blood sample on a card,
which is mailed to the maker. In a week there is a report.
An instruction booklet comes with the kit. Positive

testers get over-the-phone counseling. Negative testers hear a recorded message. Home Access® is very similar and costs $40.50 (in 1997) with an answer back in three to seven days. Both kits proved extremely accurate in their premarketing testing. At least three more self-testing kits are about to enter the market.

Testing via a hospital or commercial laboratory, or your own physician's office, may make your record open to many more individuals than anonymous or confidential testing would, possibly to your disadvantage. If a physician learns of a patient's positive HIV test, it is the physician's duty to tell the patient to inform all sexual contacts of the test result. It is also the physician's duty to bring the patient up to date on safer sex practices. For any illness, sexually transmitted or otherwise, some health professionals feel morally obligated to violate confidentiality if it is necessary to protect someone who may suffer serious harm if they remain unaware of a patient's condition.

For whatever reasons, if you decide that no one, not your doctor, not your contacts, nor anyone else, is to learn of your test result, you should have anonymous testing.

18

Summing Up

We all lead a sexual life of one kind or another, but we are not born with the knowledge we need to be able to engage in sexual activities for maximal rewards and minimal penalties. Something as simple as the appropriate use of soap and water can magnify the pleasure of the senses, foster peace of mind, and help shelter us from the trauma of sexually transmitted disease. We have to learn about sex through a broad process we call sex education.

Sex education begins at birth and is lifelong. How we dress male and female infants, the toys children are encouraged to play with, and our observation of how parents behave toward each other and toward their children are all part of the process. This book is also part of the process. It has presented a narrow view of some problem areas in basic, practical sexuality. My focus has been on a limited array of sexual health topics which, for all our vast media fascination with matters sexual, have been inadequately exposed to public scrutiny.

Not just sex but life itself presents us with countless problems. To deal with these as successfully as possible takes a great stock of acquired knowledge, a high level of maturity, sufficient self-knowledge to understand a good part of the time why we do, or react, as we do, plus insight into the basic drives of others and some appreciation of what makes them tick, as well as a supply of common sense, and some luck. Possession of an inner poise that allows for freedom to respond to situations in an emotionally appropriate way and a sense of humor always on stand-by are additional assets. All these qualities augmented by love for the partner and a sufficient level of sexual expertise empower individuals to give and receive the endless sexual riches available to us.

If we want the full measure of sexual bliss that may exist for us, we have to do our homework to become sexually educated. The risks of failing to absorb these important lessons may lead us to misery. The joys of mastering the material can be wonderful.

We all look forward to a sexual life brimming with fulfillment and pleasure. It's a shameful waste to allow minor annoyances and avoidable dangers to spoil it for us.

Glossary

Pronunciation for uncommon words is phonetically indicated. An accent mark with an "a" below it (à) between hyphens (-à-) or between letters (mànt) represents an indeterminate sound, a short *uh*-like sound, like the "a" in around or the "u" in circus.

An apostrophe after a syllable indicates the most stressed syllable in the word. A quotation mark after a syllable indicates a lesser stressing of that syllable.

Abortion. The premature termination of pregnancy before the fetus is able to live outside the uterus.

AIDS (àids). Acquired immunodeficiency syndrome is a fatal condition brought on by infection with the human immunodeficiency virus (HIV)

Amebiasis (a"-mee-ih-buy'-à-sis). The state of being infected with amebae, especially *Entamoeba histolytica*.

Antibody (an'-tih-bod"-ee). A protein produced as a protective agent against materials foreign to the body.

ARC. AIDS-Related Complex.

Asymptomatic (ay'-simp-tà-mat'-ik). Without symptoms, producing no symptoms.

Bacillary Dysentery (bas'-i-la"-ree dís-àn-ter"-ee). Dysentery is an inflammation of the intestine, particularly the colon, with abdominal pain, episodes of straining to have a bowel movement when there is no stool in the rectum, and frequent stools containing pus and blood. Bacillary dysentery refers to dysentery caused by bacilli, rodlike forms of bacteria.

Bacterial Vaginosis (bak-tee'-ree-àl vaj-i-no'-sàs). A common condition among women that may be caused by an imbalance in the bacteria located in the vagina, bacterial vaginosis is characterized by a discharge having an unpleasant odor, although in many cases the symtoms are so minor as to go undetected.

Bacterium (pl. Bacteria). A class of single-celled, vegetable microorganisms, some of which are valued for their chemical effects and some of which may cause disease.

Balanoposthitis (bal'-an-o-pos-thigh'-tis). Inflammation of the head of the penis and its foreskin.

Barrier. Any material that prevents passage, in terms of this book, primarily of germs or sperm.

Bartholin's Glands. Lubricant-producing glands just below the surface of the skin near the entrance to the vagina.

Betadine (bay'-tà-dine"). Generically known as povidone iodine, betadine is a brown liquid with germ-killing qualities.

Bidet (bi-day'). A bathroom fixture that squirts water to wash the genital and anal regions.

Biopsy. The removal of tissue from the body for gross (with the naked eye) and microscopic examination.

Calymmatobacterium Granulomatis (kah-lim"-mah-toe-bak-teer'-ee-àm gran-yu-low-ma-tis). Also known as Donovan's body, this is the name of the bacteria that cause granuloma inguinale.

Campylobacter Enteritis (kam″-pà-low-bak′-tar en-tà-reye-tis). An inflammation of the bowel (primarily the small bowel) caused by the bacillus known as *Campylobacter jejuni*.

Candidiasis (can-di-dye-à-sis). A disease state caused by *Candida albicans*, a yeastlike fungus that normally resides in the human gastrointestinal tract without complication, but becomes pathogenic when there is an imbalance or when the host becomes debilitated from other causes.

Carrier. An individual with an asymptomatic infection, or who is able to transmit the microorganism capable of causing the disease.

Caustic (caw-stik). A material that burns or destroys tissue through chemical action.

Cell. The smallest unit of living structure capable of independent existence. A cell is comprised of a microscopic mass of living matter containing a nucleus, which holds most of the cell's genetic apparatus, embedded in cytoplasm, the storehouse of most of the fuel and machinery of the cell, with the entire cell surrounded by a chemically active membrane.

Cervix. A neck, or a narrowed section, most commonly used in reference to the uterus.

Chancre (shang'-kàr). A firm, red, painless lesion, the earliest manifestation of syphilis.

Chancroid (shanq-kroid). A sexually transmitted disease caused by the bacillus *Haemophilus ducreyi.*

Chemotherapy. The use of chemicals (chemotherapeutic agents) to treat disease.

Chlamydia (klà-mid'-ee-à). A group of bacteria, capable of causing a variety of human diseases, that can only reproduce within a host's cell.

Circumcise. To surgically remove the foreskin.

Clitoris. A structure of the female situated at the most anterior of the vulva very similar to the male's penis, but smaller and lacking a passage for urine.

Coinfection. Separate, independent infections invading an individual at, or about, the same time.

Coitus. Human penile-vaginal sexual intercourse.

Contagious. Transmitted by contact with an infected person, his or her bodily fluids, or something that has touched either.

Contaminant. Something that makes dirty or impure that with which it mixes or contacts.

Contraception. The prevention of conception, that is, prevention of the initiation of a pregnancy.

Crabs. Slang for a crab (pubic) louse infestation.

Culture. To grow microorganisms in nutrient materials for the purpose of isolating organisms so that they may be identified.

Cunnilingus (kun″-à-ling′-gàs). Oral stimulation of the clitoris and vulva.

Cystitis (sis-tie′-tis). Inflammation of the urinary bladder.

Cytomegalovirus (CMV) (sigh″-toe-meg″-à-low-vye′-ras). A member of the herpes virus family that may produce a variety of syndromes frequently affecting the salivary glands and causing enlargement of the cells of various organs.

Diaphragm (die′-a-fram). A flexible metal ring covered with a dome-shaped sheet of material placed in the vagina as a contraceptive device.

Donovan's Body. See *Calymmatobacterium Granulomatis*.

Douche (doosh). A stream of water, sometimes medicated, for cleansing or therapy.

Ectopic Pregnancy. A pregnancy in which the fertilized egg implants outside the uterus.

Ejaculation. The ejection of semen.

Endometrium (en-doe-mee'-tree-àm). The mucous membrane lining of the uterus.

Enterobiasis (en''-tàr-o-beye'-à-sis). An infection with nematode worms, especially *Enterobius vermicularis*, the human pinworm.

Epidemic. A greater than normal frequency of occurrence of a disease.

Epididymis (ep''-à-did'-i-miss'). A tube located on the back of each testis which is part of the duct system involved in the production and expulsion of sperm.

Escherichia coli (E. coli) (esh''-àr-ik'-ee-à coe'-lie). Normal bacterial inhabitants of the colon capable of causing infections elsewhere in the body; the most common cause of inflammation of the female urinary bladder.

Fellatio (fà-lay'-she-o''). Oral stimulation of the penis.

Foreskin. The fold of skin covering the head of the penis or clitoris. Also known as the *prepuce*.

Fungus (pl. fungi). Any of numerous plants of the division or subkingdom *Thallophyta*, lacking chlorophyll, ranging in form from a single cell to a body mass of branched filamentous hyphae that often produce specialized fruiting bodies, and including the yeasts, molds, smuts, and mushrooms.

Gamma Globulin (gam″-a glob′-yà-làn). A preparation of proteins found in liquid human plasma containing the antibodies of normal adults.

Genital. The reproductive organs, especially those that are exposed (external).

Genital Mycoplasmas (jen′-à-tàl my″-ko-plaz′-màz). Parasitic bacterial inhabitants of the vagina and cervix, sometimes the cause of clinical infection in women and men.

Genital Warts. See *Human Papilloma Virus.*

Genitourinary (jen″-à-toe-yoor′-à-nehr-ee). Referring to the genital and urinary structures and functions.

Giardiasis (jee″-ahr-dye′-à-sis). Infection with *Giardia lamblia,* a flattened, heart-shaped protozoan that attaches itself to the mucous membranes lining the intestine.

Glans. The head of the penis and the clitoris.

Gonorrhea (gon"-à-ree'-à). A contagious, sexually transmitted inflammation of the genital mucous membrane.

Granuloma Inguinale (gran"-yà-low'-mà in"-gwàn'-ahl). A chronic, ulcer-producing, sexually transmitted, inflammatory condition primarily affecting the skin and mucous membranes of the genital region.

Hepatitis (hep"-à-tie'-tis). An inflammation of the liver usually caused by a viral infection.

Herpes (her'-peez). A family of viruses causing disease characterized by the formation of blisters on the skin and/or mucous membranes.

HIV. See **AIDS.**

Human Papilloma Virus (HPV). The virus that causes genital warts, which are cauliflowerlike growths appearing on the vulva, vagina, cervix, and other reproductive organs of both males and females. Although ordinarily benign, some types of HPV have been linked to cancers and precancers.

Hygiene. The science of health and maintaining good health.

Immunity. An ability to resist disease.

Incubation Period. The time from an infection's entry into the body to the development of the first symptoms and/or signs.

Infection. The condition in which invading microorganisms multiply in the body with varying degrees of harmful effect.

Infectious. Capable of causing infection.

Infertility. The condition of being incapable of producing a child.

Inflammation. A bodily response to infection, irritation, or injury in which an affected area becomes red, painful, and congested with blood.

Intrauterine Device (IUD). A device inserted and left in the uterus to prevent pregnancy.

–itis (eye'-tis). The suffix indicating inflammatory disease of the part of the body named in the prefix. For example, "appendicitis" is an inflammation of the appendix.

Irritation. An abnormal sensitivity, early soreness, or beginning inflammation of a part of the body.

Jock Itch. The common name for *tinea cruris.*

Kaposi's Sarcoma (kap'-o-seez sahr-ko'-mà). A malignant tumor of blood vessels frequently a component of AIDS, Kaposi's sarcoma usually appears as purple lesions on the skin, although it may also occur elsewhere in the body.

Labia Majora (lay'-bee-à mà-jor'-à). The rounded, fleshy folds that make up the outer boundaries of the vulva.

Labia Minora (mi-nor'-à). The thin, hairless, inner folds of tissue that lie between the labia majora.

Lesion (lee'-zhàn). Any abnormal structural change in the body due to injury or disease.

Lymph Node. Rounded or oval structures lying along lymph channels that remove foreign material, including microorganisms, from the lymph, a pale liquid circulating through the body consisting mainly of white blood cells and blood plasma. The nodes release lymphocytes, agents of the immune system, into the circulatory system.

Lymphocytes. See *Lymph Node.*

Lymphogranuloma Venereum (lim''-fà-gran-yà-lo'-mà và-neer'-ee-àm). A venereal infection usually caused by *Chlamydia trachomatis* characterized by a genital ulcer and enlarged lymph nodes, which eventually drain through disease-induced openings.

Masturbation. Stimulation of the genital region, usually to orgasm, other than by sexual intercourse, and particularly by oneself.

Menstruation. A discharging of bloody matter at approximately monthly intervals from the uterus of nonpregnant, reproductive-age females.

Molluscum Contagiosum (moll-us'-kum kàn-tay'-jee-o'-sum). A self-limited viral skin infection that is transmitted sexually and nonsexually.

Mononucleosis. The condition in which there are an abnormally large number of white blood cells with single nuclei in the blood.

Mucous Membrane. A membrane lining all body passages that communicate with the air, such as the respiratory and alimentary tracts, and having cells and associated glands that secrete mucus.

Nonoxynol-9. (no-nox'-i-nol). The active ingredient in many spermicides.

Nonspecific. Having no definite cause (often used in reference to infections, the source of which cannot be identified).

Os (ahss). Mouth or opening, as of the cervix.

Ovaries (o'-va-reez). In the female, a pair of reproductive glands that produce hormones and ova, the eggs.

Pap Test, Pap Smear. Most commonly, a smear taken from the surface or fluids of the cervix and adjacent vagina stained and examined microscopically for abnormal cells, including cancer cells, or for infectious agents or evidence of inflammation.

Pathological (path"-o-loj'-ik-àl). A state related to or caused by disease.

Pediculosis Pubis (pà-dik"-yà-lo'-sis pyoo'-biss). An infestation with lice, mostly just above and about the genitals.

Peritonitis (pehr"-a-toe-nigh'-tis). An inflammation of the peritoneum, the thin covering of the abdominal cavity and its contents.

Pharynx (far'-ingks). The part of the digestive tract from the back of the palate to the beginning of the esophagus (at the level of the voice box).

Pheromone (fer'-oh-moan). A chemical substance produced in animals that evokes a strong physical response in the opposite sex of the same species.

Pinworm. Pinworms are also called threadworms. They live in the human intestine.

Pneumocystis carinii (noo″-moe-sis′-tis kà-reye′-nee-eye). The causative microorganism of a specific type of pneumonia, a major cause of death in AIDS.

Prepuce (pree′-pyoos). A usually retractable fold of skin covering the head of the penis or clitoris also known as the *foreskin*.

Prophylactic (pro″-fà-lak′-tic). An agent intended to prevent disease.

Prostatitis (pros″-tà-tie′-tis). An inflammation of the prostate gland.

Protozoan (pro″-tà-zoe′-àn). A single-celled organism, the most primitive form of animal life. Some protozoa cause disease.

Pus. A thick, often yellowish liquid formed in infected tissues containing germs, white blood cells, and tissue debris.

Putrefaction (pyoo″-trà-fak′-shàn). A process of decomposition of organic matter by microorganisms in which offensive-smelling material is produced.

Rectum. The lowest part of the intestinal tract, ending at the anus.

Reiter's Syndrome. An arthritis associated with nonbacterial inflammation of the urethra or the cervix, pink eye (conjunctivitis), and skin and/or mucous membrane lesions.

Salmonella (sal"-mà-néll-à). Any of a genus of rod-shaped bacteria that cause various illnesses (such as food poisoning).

Salpingitis (sal"-pin-jeye'-tis). An inflammation of the uterine tubes.

Scabies (skay'-beez). A contagious intense itch caused by the mite, *Sarcoptes scabiei*, living as parasites in the skin. In animals other than humans, the condition is frequently called mange.

Scrotum. In most mammals, the skin-covered sac that holds the testes.

Sebaceous (si-bay'-shàs). Of, relating to, or secreting fat or fatlike substances.

Secondary Infection. An infection occurring in someone already ill in which an organism different from that causing the original illness contaminates the currently infected site.

Semen. A thick, whitish liquid produced by the male reproductive organs, a small part of which is sperm.

Sexual Hygiene. The science concerned with the preservation of sexual health and the prevention of sexual diseases.

Sexual Intercourse. Usually male-female penile-vaginal intercourse, also known as *coitus*.

Shigellosis (shih"-ghel-lo'-sis). See *bacillary dysentery*.

Smegma (smeg'-mà). A foul-smelling, pasty accumulation of dead skin cells and sebum (material produced by sebaceous glands), most prominently in the area covered by the *foreskin*.

Sperm. The mature sex cells of a male animal. See also *semen*.

Spermicide (spurm'-ih-side"). A substance capable of killing sperm.

Spirochete (speye'-row-keet"). A spiral-shaped bacterium.

STD. Sexually transmitted disease.

Superinfection. A fresh infection added to one of the same nature already present. The superinfection is usually resistant to the chemotherapeutic agents being used to treat the original infection.

Symptom. Any manifestation of disease sensed as a departure from normal.

Syndrome. A collection of signs and symptoms that characterize a particular abnormality.

Syphilis (sif'-à-lis). An acute and chronic infectious disease caused by a spirochete and transmitted by direct contact, usually through sexual intercourse.

T Cells. Any of several lymphocytes specialized particularly for activity in and control of the body's immune functions.

Tinea Cruris (tin'-ee-a croo'-ris). Ringworm of the genital region, including the inner thighs and groin.

Trichomoniasis (trik"-o-mo-neye'-à-sis). A disease caused by infection with a species of parasitic protozoa. Trichomoniasis is frequently used to refer to an acute infection resulting in vaginitis or urethritis.

Ulcer. A lesion on the surface of the skin or a mucous surface resulting from shedding of dead inflammatory tissue.

Urethra (yoo-ree'-thrà). The canal that carries urine from the bladder to outside the body.

Urethritis (yoo"-reth-reye'-tis). Inflammation of the urethra.

Uterus (yoo'-ter-as). In women, a pear-shaped muscular structure in which a fertilized egg implants and a baby develops during pregnancy.

Vaginitis (vaj"-à-neye'-tis). Inflammation of the vagina.

Venereal Disease. A contagious disease usually acquired by having sexual intercourse with an infected person.

Virus (veye'-ràs). Any of a large group of submicroscopic infectious agents that have an outside coat of protein and a core of RNA or DNA. Viruses can grow and multiply only in living cells.

Vulva. The external genitalia of the female, including the labia majora, the labia minora, and the clitoris.

Bibliography

Baldwin, Dorothy. *Understanding Male Sexual Health.* New York: Hippocrene Books, 1991.

Bechtel, Stefan. *The Practical Encyclopedia of Sex and Health: From Aphrodisiacs and Hormones to Potency, Stress, Vasectomy, and Yeast Infection.* Emmaus, Pa.: Rodale Press, 1993.

Benenson, Abram S., ed. *Control of Communicable Diseases in Man.* Washington, D.C.: American Public Health Association, 1990.

Boston Women's Health Book Collective. *The New Our Bodies, Ourselves: A Book by and for Women.* New York: Simon and Schuster, 1992.

Brackett, James. *Safe Sex: A Guide to Condoms.* Durant, Okla.: Essential Medical Information Systems, 1991.

Breitman, Patti, et al. *How to Persuade Your Lover to Use a Condom . . . And Why You Should.* Rocklin, Calif.: Prima Publishing and Communications, 1987.

Brody, Jane. *The New York Times Guide to Personal Health.* New York: Times Books, 1982.

Calderone, Mary S., and Eric W. Johnson. *The Family Book About Sexuality.* New York: Harper & Row, 1981.

Covington, Timothy R. *Sex Care: The Complete Guide to Safe and Healthy Sex.* New York: Pocket Books, 1987.

Epps, Roselyn P. and Susan C. Stewart, eds. *The Women's Complete Health Book.* New York: Delacorte Press, 1995.

Fiedler, Jean, and Hal Fiedler, Ph.D. *Be Smart about Sex: Facts for Young People.* Hillside, N.J.: Enslow Publishers, 1990.

Fenwick, Elizabeth, and Richard Walker. *How Sex Works: A Clear, Comprehensive Guide for Teenagers to Emotional, Physical, and Sexual Maturity.* London; New York: Dorling Kindersley, 1994.

The Good Health Fact Book: A Complete Question-and-Answer Guide to Getting Healthy and Staying Healthy. Pleasantville, N.Y.: Reader's Digest Association, 1992.

Holmes, King K., et al., eds. *Sexually Transmitted Diseases.* New York: McGraw-Hill, 1990.

Korte, Diana. *Every Woman's Body: Everything You Need to Know to Make Informed Choices about Your Health.* New York: Ballantine Books, 1994

Lumiere, Richard, and Stephani Cook. *Healthy Sex—and Keeping It That Way: A Complete Guide to Sexual Infections.* New York: Simon and Schuster, 1983

McCloskey, Jenny. *Your Sexual Health.* San Francisco. Halo Books, 1993.

McIlhaney, Joe S., Jr., *Safe Sex: A Doctor Explains the Realities of*

AIDS and Other STDs. Grand Rapids, Mich.: Baker Book House, 1991.

McIlvenna, Ted, ed. *The Complete Guide to Safer Sex.* Fort Lee, N.J.: Barricade Books, 1992.

MacLean, Helene, ed. *Everywoman's Health: The Complete Guide to Body and Mind.* New York: Prentice Hall Press, 1980.

The New Good Housekeeping Family Health and Medical Guide. New York: Hearst Books, 1989.

Rakel, Robert E., ed. *Conn's Current Therapy.* Philadelphia: W. B. Saunders, 1993.

Schroeder, Dirk G. *Staying Healthy in Asia, Africa, and Latin America.* Chico, Calif.: Moon Publications.

Simon, Harvey B. *Staying Well.* Boston: Houghton Mifflin, 1992.

Tierney, Lawrence M., et al., eds. *Current Medical Diagnosis and Treatment.* East Norwalk, Conn.: Appleton & Lange, 1997.

The University of California, Berkeley, Wellness Letter. *The Wellness Encyclopedia.* Boston: Houghton Mifflin, 1991.

Vargo, Marc. *The HIV Test.* New York: Pocket Books, 1992.

Westheimer, Ruth, ed. *Dr. Ruth's Encyclopedia of Sex.* New York: Continuum, 1994.

———. *Dr. Ruth's Guide to Safer Sex.* New York: Warner Books, 1992.

Whipple, Beverly, and Gina Ogden. *Safe Encounters: How Women Can Say Yes to Pleasure and No to Unsafe Sex.* New York: McGraw-Hill Book Company, 1989.

Winikoff, Beverly, Suzanne Wymelenberg, and the editors of Consumer Reports Books. *The Contraceptive Handbook: A Guide to Safe and Effective Choices.* Yonkers, N.Y.: Consumer Reports Books, 1992.

Index

peritoneum, 21, 22
peritonitis, 21, 22, 24
pharynx, 129, 141
pheromone, 17
Phthirus pubis, 88
pinworm (*see* enterobiasis)
plastic wrap, 39, 58, 64, 90, 102, 131
Pneumocystis carinii, 148, 149
posthitis, 71
pregnancy, 19, 44, 60, 67, 83, 95, 99, 145, 152, 155
  ectopic, 49, 130
  fear of, 42, 44–45
  preventing, 58, 59
  unwanted, 31, 60
prepuce (*see* foreskin)
progesterone, 22
prostate gland, 81
prostitute, prostitution, 46, 50–51, 114
protease inhibitors, 151
pubic lice, 63, 88–89
pubis, 16, 30

rectal intercourse (*see* anal [rectal] intercourse)
rectum, 29, 37, 56, 64, 83, 120, 122, 126, 129, 145

Reiter's syndrome, 72–75
rimming (*see* anilingus)
rubber glove, 39, 58, 64

Salmonella, 73, 104–105
salmonellosis, 101, 104
salpinx (uterine tube), 120
sanitary napkin (pad), 19
Sarcoptes scabiei, 86
scabies, 86–87
scrotum, 51, 85, 111, 126
sebaceous glands, 25
semen, 10, 95, 127, 139, 145
sex toys, 65, 66, 146
sexually transmitted diseases (STDs), 11–12, 28, 31, 32, 34, 35, 38, 39, 41–50, 52–53, 56, 57–58, 61–64, 66, 67, 68, 69–75, 80, 81, 86, 88, 89, 92, 93, 102, 111, 112, 113, 115, 116, 117, 121, 123, 135, 138, 140, 141, 154, 155, 157, 159
shigellosis (*see* bacillary dysentery)
"short-arm" examination, 51
showering, 26
smear, 72, 79, 84, 115, 116,